WINDY DRYDEN was born in London in 1950. He has worked in psychotherapy and counselling for over 25 years and is the author or editor of over 120 books, including *How to Accept Yourself*, and *Overcoming Envy* (both published by Sheldon Press). Dr Dryden is Professor of Psychotherapeutic Studies at Goldsmiths' College, University of London.

JACK GORDON was born in Dundee in 1921. After working for many years in a variety of management jobs he trained in Rational-Emotive Therapy, and now intends to devote his life to popularizing RET through writing and speaking.

D

Overcoming Common Problems Series

For a full list of titles please contact
Sheldon Press, Marylebone Road, London NW1 4DU

Antioxidants
Dr Robert Youngson

The Assertiveness Workbook
Joanna Gutmann

Beating the Comfort Trap
Dr Windy Dryden and Jack Gordon

Body Language
Allan Pease

Body Language in Relationships
David Cohen

Calm Down
Dr Paul Hauck

Cancer – A Family Affair
Neville Shone

The Cancer Guide for Men
Helen Beare and Neil Priddy

The Candida Diet Book
Karen Brody

Caring for Your Elderly Parent
Julia Burton-Jones

Cider Vinegar
Margaret Hills

Comfort for Depression
Janet Horwood

Considering Adoption?
Sarah Biggs

Coping Successfully with Hay Fever
Dr Robert Youngson

Coping Successfully with Pain
Neville Shone

Coping Successfully with Panic Attacks
Shirley Trickett

Coping Successfully with PMS
Karen Evennett

Coping Successfully with Prostate Problems
Rosy Reynolds

Coping Successfully with RSI
Maggie Black and Penny Gray

Coping Successfully with Your Hiatus Hernia
Dr Tom Smith

Coping Successfully with Your Irritable Bladder
Dr Jennifer Hunt

Coping Successfully with Your Irritable Bowel
Rosemary Nicol

Coping When Your Child Has Special Needs
Suzanne Askham

Coping with Anxiety and Depression
Shirley Trickett

Coping with Blushing
Dr Robert Edelmann

Coping with Bronchitis and Emphysema
Dr Tom Smith

Coping with Candida
Shirley Trickett

Coping with Chronic Fatigue
Trudie Chalder

Coping with Coeliac Disease
Karen Brody

Coping with Cystitis
Caroline Clayton

Coping with Depression and Elation
Dr Patrick McKeon

Coping with Eczema
Dr Robert Youngson

Coping with Endometriosis
Jo Mears

Coping with Epilepsy
Fiona Marshall and
Dr Pamela Crawford

Coping with Fibroids
Mary-Claire Mason

Coping with Gallstones
Dr Joan Gomez

Coping with Headaches and Migraine
Shirley Trickett

Coping with a Hernia
Dr David Delvin

Coping with Long-Term Illness
Barbara Baker

Coping with the Menopause
Janet Horwood

Coping with Psoriasis
Professor Ronald Marks

Coping with Rheumatism and Arthritis
Dr Robert Youngson

Overcoming Common Problems Series

Overcoming Common Problems Series

Overcoming Common Problems

THINK YOUR WAY TO HAPPINESS

Dr Windy Dryden and
Jack Gordon

sheldon **PRESS**

First published in Great Britain 1990 by
Sheldon Press, 1 Marylebone Road, London NW1 4DU

Ninth impression 2002

British Library Cataloguing in Publication Data

A catalogue record for this book is available from the British Library

ISBN 0–85969–603–0

Typeset by Deltatype Ltd, Ellesmere Port, Cheshire
Printed and bound in Great Britain by
Biddles Ltd, www.biddles.co.uk

Contents

Foreword

What is the value of a book on emotional health? Too many people are of the opinion that emotional problems always require months or even years of in-depth therapy. The image of Freud sitting at the head of his couch while he listens to his patients dig up the dark secrets of their past is a very popular one, but this notion that a therapist is always necessary if we are to gain control of our lives is not only exaggerated, it is downright false. What might have been fairly accurate decades ago is simply no longer true.

Psychology today has moved miles beyond Freud. Counselling people for their emotional disturbances no longer calls for a couch, nor daily sessions, and normally takes no more than a few to about twenty sessions. However, even more changes, fundamental changes in the philosophy behind therapy, have also appeared.

For example, everyday emotional problems such as depression, anger, anxiety, jealousy, and excessive passivity are no longer thought of as physical and medical problems most of the time. Some of these disorders can, of course, be the result of bodily organs not functioning smoothly, but the vast majority of the complaints people seek counselling for are psychological in nature. That is to say, most emotional problems are learned. They are bad habits, if you will, which we all learned as we grew up. We were *taught* how to feel guilty, depressed, angry, and how to worry ourselves to the point that we bite our nails, develop insomnia, or are afraid to leave our homes.

Strange as this may sound, it is the best explanation we have today of how neurotic emotions are created. Our parents, teachers, and friends have all learned the same self-defeating habits the same way we did. In fact, they taught them to us and we passed them on to our friends and children.

This is only the beginning of the changes in our understanding of disturbed behaviours. For if these are habits which we learn then how do we change them? With education, obviously. I insist people get angry because they were taught to by their families. They continue to have tantrums all their lives unless someone teaches them how not to get angry. How can this be accomplished? Why, by getting lessons from a teacher who knows how anger is created. Who is this teacher? The counsellor. We also call them psychotherapists and we refer to their work as therapy. When examined objectively we cannot deny that people today who seek help for emotional and interpersonal difficulties

1

are in fact not sick, they just need to learn. They don't need therapy, they need education. They don't usually need to see a medical doctor, they need an educator or a tutor who can teach them in his or her classroom (not clinic) a lesson in the basics of human behaviour.

When viewed in this manner we can achieve results the likes of which the earlier psychotherapists would have envied. True, some emotional conditions will always be so severe that education alone will not help. For them, medical help is indispensable. The vast majority of people who seek counselling, however, need no such heroic methods. They need to learn how they upset themselves and how they can unupset themselves.

This brings me to the purpose of my writing a foreword to a book on psychology. What is more natural to the educational process than textbooks? Is this not a time-honoured method of educating people on all manner of subjects from instruction in foreign languages to playing a musical instrument? Then why should it be surprising that educational materials should not be used in teaching people principles in emotional health? Psychology is no different from geography. Both can be taught through tutoring or classroom techniques, and both can utilize books as tools to maximize education.

If you have reservations about the place of bibliotherapy (therapy through the study of pertinent books) in the counselling process, then let me give you illustrations of other, but similar, educational tools to teach people to be psychologically healthy.

For years, I have readily referred my own clients to the best books on Cognitive-Behaviour Therapy, of which Rational-Emotive Therapy is the best model. In fact, I have written fourteen books to help improve their gains from counselling. I believe I am being objective when I report to you that bibliotherapy has earned a most respected niche in the list of techniques we counsellors have at our disposal. A book, after all, has the great advantage of being easily reread. It's there to be studied at leisure, to be put aside and picked up later to help you grasp a different concept. It cannot answer all your questions, of course. This is why bibliotherapy is more efficient in conjunction with counselling. However, leaving this shortcoming aside, it is important to impart knowledge to a client before, during or after therapy. The truth is always the truth and usually helps people manage their lives better.

Audio tapes offer similar advantages. Some persons simply dislike reading and prefer the auditory route. Whether through visual or auditory channels, the common element between tapes and books is the educational one. I have also written a weekly newspaper column and am often informed by readers how helpful some of my columns have been.

2

Then there is telephone therapy. For years I have counselled people from Mexico to Canada, from California to London, people whom I have never seen but who were nevertheless able to learn how to understand themselves and others.

Finally, letter writing has also succeeded in a number of instances. My mail from India, Australia, or Europe is always answered, and in a few instances has turned into a correspondence over a period of months or years with distinctly beneficial results.

Having made these observations, I trust you will have faith in the efficiency of books to teach you better emotional control.

What kind of book is appropriate for you? Whether this is your first popular book in self-help psychology or your tenth, it should have certain qualities for it to be worthy of recommendation.

(1) It must be written for the layman. That means that complex psychological ideas must be translated into the language of the person in the street. That's not always easily done. Some writers have an irresistible temptation to flaunt their professional vocabularies and go over the heads of their frustrated readers. Do not trouble yourself to read books which do not respect your right *not* to know the field as well as the authors do.

(2) It must be written by qualified professional psychologists, psychiatrists, or social workers. Not only should the authors have the proper degrees but they must also have extensive experience as psychotherapists. Doctor Windy Dryden (whom I had the pleasure of meeting in August 1988 in London) and Jack Gordon (whom I also personally know) are both recognized as highly qualified practitioners of RET.

(3) It must be practical. A self- help book had better be just that – a self-help book – or it's a fake. That doesn't mean it will cure all the reader's problems. No book has ever been able to come even close to such a goal. However, among the self-help books you should read is one which gives you the fundamentals in self-help techniques. It focuses on those issues which trouble us the most, especially how we get upset and what to do about it. In fact, a proper book of this sort never loses sight of that target.

(4) Summaries, either throughout the book or at its end, help the student review what has been taught and thereby offers a refresher course. This book has such summaries at the end of each chapter. I have read them and found them helpful – just as I had expected.

(5) The book must deal with the most common emotional problems, not the extraordinary ones. This surely includes precisely those

3

disorders Windy Dryden and Jack Gordon devote most of their pages to. Depression, of course, has to be included. I have called it the most painful emotion, and the authors have very kindly mentioned the views on depression I offered in my book *Depression,* published by Sheldon Press. They also include the most dangerous emotion, anger, and explain how we make ourselves furious, and how to correct that condition so that it is no more dangerous than an irritation. Anxiety and worry, self-discipline, shame, shyness, and guilt are also all dealt with at their basic and fundamental levels.

Can you believe that it is possible to control these savage and crippling behaviours to a degree where anger is reduced to annoyance, guilt to regret and fear to curiosity? Our disturbances will not be eliminated totally and forever – that would leave us behaving like robots. No, we will always respond to frustrations as humans, not machines – but let us do this to an appropriate degree, not to a neurotic degree.

That is what this book and others like it strive for. We want more control over ourselves, and we want to get along with others better. Fortunately these are skills psychology is able to teach better today than ever before. And one of the best places to start this educational process is to read a book which deals with the fundamentals in a readable style. I am pleased to announce that such a book is now available. Its title is *Think Your Way to Happiness*. Its authors are Dr Windy Dryden and Jack Gordon. The publisher is Sheldon Press and it is my pleasure to speak on their behalf.

Dr Paul A. Hauck
Rock Island, Illinois

1
Basic Ideas

If you ask people what kinds of things really upset them, you will get a great variety of answers. Some of the more typical responses you will hear go something like this:

(1) 'It's my husband's constant bellyaching that upsets me. It makes me really mad! It goes on and on, day in and day out. Nothing I ever do seems to be right for him.'

(2) 'Our teenage daughter is just impossible. She makes us so angry! She's out every night, sometimes till after twelve. Some mornings we can hardly get her up in time to get to work. And she never does a thing in the house to help. Her room is like a pigsty but all she does is roam around all day with her personal stereo on. She hears that alright but she never seems to hear anything we say to her.'

(3) 'My wife just uses this house as a dormitory. She's out every night, meetings here, meetings there. At weekends she's playing golf with her friends or business partners. I never see her. I feel so lonely and worried!'

(4) 'It's everything! The state of the world today, everything's going downhill. Violence, violence everywhere. And all those starving millions you read about and see on the TV news. I get so depressed just listening to it all.'

You could no doubt think of a few things yourself. Two of our clients have even insisted that it is the weather that makes them feel so depressed!

Yet every one of these 'explanations' people offer to explain their emotional upset is wrong! We are not saying that these events in people's lives don't happen. Of course they happen. There are real problems and hassles in virtually everyone's lives. Relationship problems, serious illnesses and traffic accidents are daily occurrences. And many parts of the world *are* in a pretty grim state. 'Alright, then', we can hear you say. 'If none of the situations you described cause us to get really upset, would you mind telling us just what *does* upset us?' A good question, and one we will now answer as clearly as we can.

The examples we quoted of problem situations people tell us are the causes of their troubled emotions were chosen to illustrate a very important point, namely, that almost everyone believes that emotional tensions are the direct result of stressful events which confront us, or of unpleasant situations in which we find ourselves. In other words, virtually all of us believe that external happenings *make* us upset, that our feelings of rage, despair or self-pity stem directly from those obnoxious situations and there is nothing we can do about it except to change the situation or get away from it. Up to a point this is a fairly common-sense view. If a sharp knife can cause physical pain, then sharp, cutting words should surely cause some emotional pain – like intense shame or guilt, for example. Up to a point it sounds logical. All of us at some time or other have been on the receiving end of some sarcastic or belittling words and have felt so 'put down' that we were unable to think of any adequate response.

Nevertheless, this popular view fails to explain, as we shall demonstrate, the reasons for emotional distress. An unfortunate event which may trigger off an anxiety attack in you one day, may leave you relatively unaffected on another day even if the external circumstances are the same in each instance. And isn't it common knowledge that while John may be 'bowled over' by some activating circumstance, like being rejected on a date by a particularly attractive member of the opposite sex, Laurence will take the same experience in his stride?

The core of emotional disturbance

Over the past few years a considerable amount of research by psychologists and practitioners in mental health disciplines has thrown light on how emotional turmoil is created and how it can be tackled and eliminated. While psychoanalytic practitioners attempted to locate the sources of emotional disturbance in childhood conflicts with parental figures, more recently many psychotherapists, including ourselves, have espoused the model of human emotional disturbance first devised and developed by Dr Albert Ellis, an American clinical psychologist, in 1955. Known as the A-B-C model of emotional disturbance, it forms the core of a system of psychotherapy created by Ellis called Rational-Emotive Therapy, or RET for short. According to the A-B-C theory, mental suffering does not come directly from the problems that beset us but from the irrational and false notions we have about them. Thus to overcome your upsetting feelings and regain your emotional equilibrium you need to identify the false ideas which generate the disturbed feelings and then to uproot them by the rigorous application of logic and reason until you convince yourself of the irrationality of your previously held ideas. Provided you subsequently behave in accordance with your new, more rational, ideas, your disturbed emotions will fade and become replaced by more healthy and appropriate responses. To illustrate what we mean by these remarks let us take as an example a fairly common experience.

You have seen a job advertised that you would very much like to be accepted for. You consider yourself well qualified to apply for the post. It is the job you have been waiting for – interesting, challenging, well paid and with excellent prospects for further advancement. You apply, you are interviewed, and you are rejected. In terms of the A-B-C model, A, what we call the *activating event*, stands for the rejection. Let's assume you feel terribly depressed. We call that the *emotional consequence* (C), which stands for your feelings and actions. You have just been rejected at point A for this wonderful job, and at point C you are feeling really depressed. You have lost your appetite, you feel listless and when your friends call round to ask you to join them in some social activity, your response is: 'Oh, what's the use, I've no energy. Just go without me.' The common-sense view would be that you went after a great job and you failed to land it and, of course, that made you depressed. Most people would believe that. And they'd be wrong! No, A did not cause C. Your depression stems from point B. B stands for your belief system, in this instance, your beliefs about the job and about yourself in relation to the job. These beliefs, which consist primarily of evaluations and appraisals, are of two kinds – a rational set and an irrational set. Let's take the rational beliefs first. Remember, these are the sane beliefs you hold about being rejected for the job. They will usually be of the order: 'I don't like being rejected because it has real disadvantages. I wanted to be accepted but was rejected and that is certainly unfortunate and very frustrating.' If you are asked to prove your statement, you can easily present hard facts, which anyone else can check, to show that it *is* unfortunate that you've been rejected. Thus, you can show that rejection leads to fewer chances of job advancement, to lower future income, less interesting work, and so on. You can show that the inconvenient consequences of rejection hardly justify opening the champagne. It is quite inappropriate for you to feel joyous or delighted, and most appropriate to feel sorrowful, regretful, frustrated and even annoyed. Your feelings of sorrow and frustration are appropriate because it is hardly appropriate to feel glad and unfrustrated when you are truly frustrated and inconvenienced. Moreover, your feelings of annoyance may actually stimulate you to doing something constructive to improve your performance on interviews the next time round. 'So far, so good!' we can hear you say. 'But you have just painted a picture of someone feeling deeply depressed. Where does that fit in?' Right! Let's go back to the point we made about your beliefs consisting of two kinds: a set of rational thoughts about the job rejection and a set of irrational thoughts or evaluations about the job rejection. Now we showed you that if your thoughts about the job rejection consisted of *only* rational beliefs, the feelings you would

7

experience as a result of those sane, reality-based thoughts would amount to strong disappointment. They would not send you into an acute depression. Your depression would be created by the other set of beliefs – the irrational beliefs which are essentially false notions and unprovable assumptions with no basis in reality. Typically, your irrational beliefs would be of the order: 'I *can't stand* being turned down! It's awful, horrible and catastrophic for me not to have been accepted! I *absolutely should* have been accepted rather than rejected with all my qualifications and the fact that I was not accepted proves that either I am *no good* or that my interviewer was too biased against me from the start, the rotten so-and-so!' If you convince yourself of these unrealistic notions and unprovable assumptions you will almost certainly create in yourself highly upsetting feelings such as depression, shame and hostility. Remember, the rational beliefs we alluded to above are the beliefs you *can* prove to be valid. You can logically show them to be sustainable convictions. They are reality-based.

Look for and dispute your 'shoulds' and 'musts'

In this book we shall show you how various upsetting emotions and self-defeating behaviours are created by the false or mistaken perceptions people have of reality, together with the grandiose beliefs of what *must* be and *absolutely should* be the case. We will also teach you not only how to recognize those unrealistic ideas and demands which lie at the root of emotional disturbance but also how to challenge, dispute and uproot them so that you can reduce or eliminate your poor emotional responses and replace them with more appropriate, less self-defeating patterns of feeling and behaviour. Returning to the depression we took as an example of what might happen to someone who had been rejected following a job interview, let us see how we would dispute and rip up the irrational views which are creating and sustaining the depression.

'*I can't stand being turned down!*' What does that mean? That you will literally fall apart? If you think about it you will see that this is an example of circular thinking. First, you *think* you can't stand being rejected. Second, you think you can't stand it because you *decide* not to stand it. And if you think and decide you can't stand being rejected, you will *feel* as if you can't stand it. As long as you are alive and breathing you can stand anything! Another unfortunate meaning of 'I can't stand it' is the often unspoken conviction that 'I won't ever have any happiness again'. You are more likely to jump to that conclusion following a rejection by someone you had, or would like to have had, a close relationship with, rather than after being unsuccessful in a job interview. But whatever the circumstances, your belief that you can *never* have happiness again is as devoid of rational supporting evidence as is your belief that being passed over for promotion or failing to be successful in an important job interview is a virtual catastrophe. Can you foresee the future? How could you prove to yourself that you could never, under any circumstances, experience happiness again? If you maintain you can never have any happiness again, you are probably using that belief as a justification for feeling sorry for yourself rather than taking a sensible view of your future prospects. We shall be looking into self-pity a little later. Right now, short of the certainty of facing execution in the morning, you have as much chance of finding happiness some time in the future as anyone else. As we pointed out to you before, you can only feel you are doomed to a life of unhappiness if you *think* you are. So, question your assumptions, look for the evidence. Where are the *facts* that prove incontrovertibly that you can never be happy again? If you find any, let us know; you'll become famous overnight!

'It's awful, horrible and catastrophic for me not to have been accepted.' Where is the evidence that being rejected is truly a catastrophe? You *feel* it is awful and horrible because you *think* it is awful and horrible to be rejected. But ask yourself what these words 'awful' and 'horrible' really mean. They mean, first, that it is inconvenient for you not to have been accepted. You have already proved that by referring us to your rational beliefs. We accept that. It *is* extremely inconvenient to be rejected for a job you had set your mind on winning. But when you use words like 'awful' and 'horrible' or 'catastrophic' aren't you going over the top and virtually demanding that you *should* not, *ought* not, *must* not be inconvenienced? But can you prove why anything must or should not exist? If you are inconvenienced, you are inconvenienced. Hard luck! 'What I want to exist *must* exist! When I want a job I'm being interviewed for, I *should* get it!' With godlike demands like these underlying your thinking how can you *not* feel emotionally disturbed when life does not go along with your demands? – as it frequently won't!

Accept yourself and others as fallible

In similar vein, we would go on to tackle your conviction that you are no good because you failed the interview and/or that your interviewer was biased against you and was really a louse who should never have been allowed on the panel and would have been better employed peeling potatoes. We would show you that just because you failed a job interview you are not a worthless person, just one who happens to lack particular qualities deemed necessary for a particular job by that interviewer. That may, or may not, be true. It may be that your interviewer was deficient in certain interviewing skills and failed to ascertain your true capabilities. Tough! But just as you are not a worthless person because you (presumably) lacked the ability or experience or whatever they were looking for at the interview, by the same token neither is the interviewer a bad person because he (presumably) lacked the skills required of a good interviewer; he is only a human being with certain definite limitations. Like you, he has good and bad traits, performs well in some activities and does badly or less well in others. Neither he nor you can be given a global rating; you are neither 'good' nor 'bad'. All of us are fallible human beings. For that reason it would be better if you did not try to rate or measure your entire being, your total self, at all. By all means attempt to improve your performance on various activities, or to alter certain traits you wish to improve. If you simply accept yourself unconditionally you will not only save yourself needless anxiety but be better able to change the things you can change and calmly accept those things which you cannot change.

For the moment we will leave the techniques of identifying and disputing the ideas underlying emotional disturbance for more detailed consideration in later chapters, and summarize what we have learned so far.

The A-B-C of emotional disturbance

First, emotional problems such as anxiety or depression are not caused by some external event that has happened or is likely to happen to us, but by the faulty beliefs we have about the feared event. Our emotional distress comes not from events in the real world but from the incorrect, over-generalized and irrational ideas and evaluations we hold *about* these events. Your thinking, your feeling and your behaviour are all interrelated. They all influence each other. You feel as you think and your thinking is in turn influenced by your feeling and behaviour.

To help us conceptualize a given problem we use the A-B-C model as an approach to human personality and its disturbance. Here, A stands for the activating event or experience. The upsetting emotions and self-defeating behaviours are labelled C and include the individual's feelings of anxiety or depression, worthlessness and so on. When you have an emotional or behavioural problem begin by focusing on C, the emotional and behavioural consequences and realize that an activating experience (A) in the outside world does not, and cannot, cause or create any feeling or behavioural consequences (C). For if it did, virtually everyone who gets rejected, for example, would have to feel the same emotional and behavioural reactions. Since this is hardly likely to be true, C is really caused by something that occurs between A and C. We call this B, the individual's belief system. You can think of B as a collection of core values and beliefs which you hold about yourself and the world and which make up a framework or set of reference points from which you habitually judge and react to events and experiences happening in the world.

Why think rationally?

The reason for trying to distinguish the rational from the irrational components in our thinking is not that we favour the rational *per se*. We advocate rational thinking because it helps promote human happiness. If we didn't believe that to survive happily in this world and to relate intimately to a few selected others were sensible goals of living we would scarcely bother to encourage and promote rational ways of living, either for ourselves or for others. Not that you have to select happiness as your goal in this, your one chance at life on earth. You could don a hair shirt, live in the desert and choose to suffer for the rest of your life. If that was your goal we could teach you how to suffer even more efficiently! But because we choose to follow rational dictates of living, our goals are to minimize human suffering and maximize human well-being. We, the authors of this book, want to help create a saner, happier world because that is the kind of world we prefer to live in. Through our teachings we believe and hope we can help a significant number of our fellow men and women lead less self-defeating and more self-fulfilling lives. We are not, however, aiming to help you become perfectly rational. Perfect rationality – like a perfect world – is a myth. It doesn't exist. Nevertheless, we hope you can profit from this book. Any reasonably intelligent person can learn to apply the principles of rational thinking, as set out in this book, to his or her own problems of living.

Think – and act!

But a word of warning! Merely reading and agreeing with what we say isn't going to do you much good. Unless you are really convinced of the truth of what we shall try to teach you, and unless you follow through by *acting* and practising new patterns of behaviour which reflect the new more rational philosophy you are trying to acquire, then all the reading in the world will be of little benefit. The philosophy we espouse and will teach you in later chapters may *sound* easy, but it isn't! To get the full benefit from it requires lots of action, hard work and self-discipline. Even when you are convinced that what we write is true, don't take our word for it! Think, really think about it. Find out for yourself if it is true and why. Merely parroting a few rational ideas to yourself and your friends will hardly scratch the surface. Many of the irrational ideas you currently hold are ideas you believe in strongly. You have held them for quite some time and they have become established. It follows that if you want to rid yourself of those faulty ideas and demands that are presently sustaining your troubled feelings and behaviour, then it would be better for you to work hard and consistently at undermining your irrational ideas and replacing them with more realistic ones— ideas that will lead to healthier emotions and behaviour.

The three major irrational beliefs

In subsequent chapters you will learn that most emotional difficulties spring from at least one – but more usually several – unsustainable ideas that people impose upon themselves. All those beliefs are forms of absolutism. They consist of unqualified demands and needs, instead of preferences and desires. Consequently, they have nothing to do with reality. Over the past few years three major irrational beliefs have been found to be at the root of most emotional disturbance:

(1) 'Because it would be highly preferable if I were outstandingly competent and/or loved by significant others, I absolutely should and must be. It is awful when I am not and I am therefore a worthless individual.'

(2) 'Because it is highly desirable that others treat me considerately and fairly, they absolutely should and must do so and they are rotten people who deserve to be utterly condemned when they do not.'

(3) 'Because it is preferable that I experience pleasure rather than pain, the world absolutely must arrange this and life is horrible, and I can't bear it, when the world does not.'

These three fundamental irrational beliefs and the many ideas that stem from them are the main factors underlying virtually all neurosis and character disorder. Although they may, in turn, have their own origins, unlike psychoanalysis we do not think that probing into and discovering the original causes of an individual's irrational beliefs will prove exceptionally helpful. For even if you are led to discover how you first became upset, that insight alone will not help you overcome your

12

upset now. You still, after you get this information, have to change your old conviction which you still carry round with you; and you can do this whether or not you understand how it originated. It is possible that knowing about the origin will *help* you change the ideas that caused you to feel upset long ago when you were a child. Your awareness of how your present upset feeling stems from the past, plus the realization that you are now grown up and no longer a vulnerable child, may be the first step in motivating you to change. But in the last analysis, and whether or not you ever discover how you originally became upset, it is not the original events at point A (such as your mother's or father's rejection of you) that makes you upset today at point C (at the thought of being rejected). No, it is your continued reiteration to yourself of the beliefs you formed in response to these events at point B that makes you upset. You make and keep yourself disturbed by being the kind of individual who finds it easy to do exactly these things, like all of us. If we were a different kind of being – if, when we were young, for example, we possessed the thinking ability and critical capacity of an adult to be sceptical of anything that was told to us – it is highly unlikely that the external events and parental influences that occur in childhood or later life would cause us to be overly concerned about rejection or anything else. In short, what is important is your acknowledgement that, regardless of whatever emotional traumas you may have experienced as a child, you can overcome the emotional difficulties you experience *now* by persistently challenging the irrational beliefs which underpin your problems and replacing your irrational beliefs with a sounder, reality-based philosophy. In the following chapters we shall attempt to show you in detail exactly how to go about achieving this.

Conclusion

To conclude this introductory chapter, we would make one or two important points. 'Rational' in our therapeutic system does not mean unemotional. Life is such that you may legitimately feel sad or annoyed (as when things don't go your way) as well as joyful or even ecstatic when they do. The more determined you are to be self-accepting and happiness-orientated by working with your brain and other faculties, the more emotional and the more in touch with your feelings you will tend to be. The techniques we use in Rational-Emotive Therapy (RET) and which we present in this book are designed to do more than change behaviour and help you *feel* better. They are also used to change your basic philosophies and to give you the specific means of changing these philosophies again and again if need be, until you rarely revert to self-sabotaging feelings and actions. As we have already pointed out, RET is no miracle cure. It requires a considerable amount of work and practice on your part. There are no sudden insights, no magic cures. If you work, it will enable you to understand yourself and others better and to react appropriately to life's ups and downs. You will obtain more control over your emotions and help yourself to become more creative, to enjoy life more, and to be better able to fulfil your potential.

SUMMARY POINTS FOR CHAPTER 1

The main points to be picked up from this chapter are these:

(1) You feel as you think. In fact, your feelings, your behaviour and your thinking are all interrelated. External events, such as being rejected, or experiencing some other misfortune, may contribute to your emotional response, but they do not *cause* it. In the main, you create your own feelings by the way you think about and evaluate whatever you perceive is happening to you.

(2) Whether your feelings and behaviour in response to some event in your life are appropriate and helpful, or inappropriate and self-defeating, depends on whether your beliefs about the event are rational or irrational. Rational beliefs are reality-based, beliefs you can logically demonstrate are sustainable convictions. Irrational beliefs, by contrast, consist of unrealistic notions and unprovable assumptions, embedded in some form of absolutistic demand.

(3) The A-B-C model of emotional disturbance is a quick and effective technique for conceptualizing your emotional problems and for helping you to identify and uproot the irrational components of your belief system which create and sustain upsetting emotions and self-defeating behaviours.

(4) If you are currently experiencing an emotional problem, such as anger or anxiety, for example, regardless of how you may have acquired your problem originally, you may assume that the reason why it continues to bother you is that deep down you still believe the irrational ideas which created the problem in the first place.

(5) Three major irrational ideas constitute the core of virtually all emotional disturbance:

    (a) 'Because it would be highly preferable if I were outstandingly competent and/or loved by significant others, I *must* do well and/or win the love and approval of those others (and it's awful and I'm no good if I don't).

    (b) 'You and others must treat me fairly and considerately (and if you don't, you are all rotten people who deserve to be condemned).'

(c) 'Because I prefer pleasure to pain, the world must give me what I want quickly and easily (and when the world doesn't arrange this, it's awful and I can't stand it).'

(6) We advocate rational thinking because it promotes human survival in the world and furthers personal happiness and human well-being.

(7) To obtain the full benefit from the RET philosophy we teach will require from you practice, action, hard work and self-discipline.

2

Anxiety and Worry

Anxiety and worry, the inseparable twins! There are worse things you can suffer from but anxiety and worry are among the commonest problems people seek help for. Why is this? First, anxiety and worry are closely related to fear. Fear can be a very strong emotion and there are good biological reasons for it. Our early ancestors probably had a very highly developed sense of fear because their survival frequently depended on their ability to sense danger and to take whatever action seemed most appropriate – fight or flight. We might also imagine circumstances in which our ancestors experienced what we would call 'anxiety', a vague feeling of unease or threat from some source which might be dangerous but which was not directly perceived as an immediate danger. The sound of a twig snapping suddenly in the middle of the night might be just a small animal or bird; or it might signal the presence of a hungry leopard stealthily seeking a meal. Nine times out of ten it might be nothing to cause alarm. But how could they be sure? Those who chose to get away fast would lose a night's sleep, perhaps for nothing, but they stood a better chance of passing on their genes than those others who decided to take a chance and go back to sleep!

Today, unless we choose to spend some of our lives exploring jungles or other wild places, our fears derive from the hazards of living in the latter part of the twentieth century. We may not have quite so many threats and potential threats to our lives as primitive man faced in his shorter lifespan (although this is debatable), but we make up for our lack of fear of being eaten alive by torturing ourselves with self-inflicted anxiety and worry.

Let's take a look now at what we mean by fear and anxiety.

Fear versus anxiety

When you perceive something as immediately threatening or dangerous, or anticipate that it will be in the immediate future, such as someone threatening you with a knife or gun, you will experience *fear*. That fear will normally motivate you to do something to protect yourself. The emotion will stimulate the level of adrenalin in your bloodstream which in turn will raise your blood glucose level to increase your alertness in response to the emergency. In other words, fear is normally self-protecting. If you were not appropriately fearful of

16

the many hazards to life and limb that you will normally encounter during an average lifetime the chances are you wouldn't have an average lifetime: if you had no fear whatsoever you would surely die pretty soon after you were born. You would lean too far out of windows or walk across a busy street regardless of the vehicles speeding by, and do many other things that would ensure your early demise. You can, of course, become *too* afraid, not only of real dangers and threats, but of just about anything. If that happens to you, then you have crossed over the borderline separating fear from anxiety.

Anxiety is the feeling you experience when you are unduly *over*-concerned about the possibility of some dreaded event happening in the future over which you have no control and which, if it occurred, would be rated by you as 'terrible', or which would reveal you as a totally inadequate person in your own mind. You can define anxiety also as a feeling of threat from a cause which you are presently unaware of but which is liable to erupt when you least expect it and reveal you to all and sundry (especially yourself!) as an incompetent fool or laughing stock. This type of anxiety frequently occurs in social situations. One example is a man who knows he can sometimes be a bit clumsy at table and imagines the 'horror' of a scenario in which he is the guest at a 'posh' dinner party where, after filling his lady companion's wine glass, he upsets the glass as he replaces the bottle on the table and spills the entire contents of the glass on her lap. Another example is the woman who buys herself an expensive new dress to wear at a wedding reception and worries herself for days before the event by imagining the 'horror' of turning up at the reception only to meet another woman there who is wearing exactly the same dress. You can probably imagine your own anxiety-creating 'situations', although we hope you will have realized by now that it isn't the situation itself that creates your anxiety, but the things you tell yourself *about* the situation. Thus, virtually every time you experience this kind of 'social anxiety' you are thinking, 'What if . . .' and, 'Wouldn't it be *awful* if such-and-such were to happen and people were to think badly of me?'

How we make ourselves anxious

As it happens, not all the anxiety you might experience arises from your self-deprecating thoughts at the possibility of some personal weakness or failure being publicly revealed. A second common form of anxiety springs from a philosophy held by many, indeed most people, which we call Low Frustration Tolerance, or LFT for short. You will be coming across LFT quite a few times as you read through this book because a good deal of emotional disturbance is generated by LFT. The basic idea underlying LFT is this: 'Life should be easy and go the way I want without too much trouble or annoyance; and if it doesn't, it's awful and I can't *stand* it.' If you hold to this idea, you are in the 'comfort trap'. Typical variations of this idea are, 'I must feel good', 'I mustn't feel anxious', 'I must always feel cool, calm, and collected'. If you subscribe to this thinking, and given the fact that you will begin to feel discomfort almost as soon as you think these thoughts, an anxiety attack will be the likely result. You can even become anxious about being anxious!

At this point, some of you may say: 'But surely it's normal to be anxious about some things in life? What about being killed in a car crash, for example? You read about people being killed or seriously injured every day. You can hardly set out on a journey these days, especially on those overcrowded motorways, without feeling anxious about getting back in one piece.' To which we would reply: 'Yes, it is normal in the sense of being statistically common for most people to feel anxious in those circumstances you've just described. Most people, probably all of us, have at some time or other in our lives felt anxiety in these or similar situations. But the fact that something commonly occurs doesn't mean that it has to occur or that it is desirable for it to occur. Not so long ago, most males in our society smoked cigarettes. Nowadays, as a result of changing perceptions, very many fewer males smoke cigarettes.' If we could show you how to minimize or eliminate your anxiety without abandoning your legitimate fear of life-threatening situations and how to distinguish between the two, we would bet that most people would think they had got a good deal. After all, nobody enjoys being anxious. You may at times even receive sympathy from friends who will go out of their way to find you alternative means of transport if they know how anxious you become at the prospect of being driven on a motorway to your destination. You may find your friends' sympathy gratifying but do you really want to spend the rest of your life living under a cloud of anxiety? The trouble is, as we have pointed out, that anxiety can easily become self-perpetuating. You become anxious about being anxious which becomes a vicious circle from which you find it difficult to escape. Also, it doesn't help that the reason why people find it easy to become anxious about virtually anything in life is that we have an innate predisposition to make ourselves anxious. We humans are highly suggestible animals; we are prone to exaggerate the significance of the various things that happen to us in life. While it is possible that man's possession of a high degree of suggestibility and anxiety may have had positive survival value during his long evolutionary history, he can get along with himself and others much better today when he becomes more rational, or more *intelligently* suggestible. So, let's get back to basics, to the A-B-C model we introduced you to in Chapter 1, and see if we can figure out how to retain a healthy rational concern for our safety and general well-being, while doing away with irrational fear or over-concern which leads to life-eroding anxiety.

If you have followed this A-B-C model of emotional disturbance, you should have no difficulty in understanding how you can conduct an examination of your anxiety- creating ideas. Once you admit that it is your own ideas that are making and keeping you over-concerned about the dangers of motorway driving or anything else, you can stop and examine these ideas. Let us take a specific example of one common type of anxiety.

A case of anxiety

Angela is a presentable woman of average intelligence who is terribly afraid of driving on motorways. She is a competent driver and drives carefully at all times. But Angela has convinced herself that driving on motorways is highly dangerous and that if she tried it she would lose control and some terrifying accident would result. So Angela refrains from driving on motorways and restricts herself to driving on quiet country roads near her home, and then only in good daylight. It happens that Angela now lives some distance away from her family, whom she adores and loves to visit frequently. However, as a consequence of her self-imposed restrictions on motorway driving, Angela puts herself, and her family, to a considerable amount of inconvenience when she travels to visit them because the only way she can travel to where they live is to take the train; and public transport is somewhat infrequent in Angela's part of the country. She could, of course, theoretically drive herself to where her relations live, or even take a bus, but that would mean using a motorway – and that's out as far as Angela is concerned! It transpires after some questioning of Angela's attitude to life that Angela's real problem is an inordinate fear of death. 'I'm not old,' she exclaims, 'I can't stand the thought of being killed in some crash and never again seeing my dear family whom I love so much. I'm determined to spend lots and lots more time with them and so I'm not taking any chances with my life.'

In terms of the A-B-C model, point A stands for the possibility of an accident leading to serious injury or death. At point C, Angela feels dread at the thought of never seeing her family again. Angela's dread of being involved in a possible fatality on the roads springs from her beliefs about the feared event. At point B she is telling herself: 'Wouldn't it be *awful* if my life were cut short before I've really had time to enjoy my family now that they have left home and are grown up! I can't stand the thought of being prevented from having what I've worked so hard for, and what I think I deserve. I *must* have at least another twenty years of life ahead of me to enjoy my family or else life isn't really worth living!'

Let us look now more closely at what Angela is telling herself about the possibility of her being incapacitated if she risked driving, or being driven, on motorways. Concern, if you think about it, is quite different from over-concern. If you had no concern or rational fear about the possibility of being involved in an accident whenever you drove on motorways, you might seriously damage your vehicle and maybe those of other drivers. Alert concentration on the process of driving and the road condition at all times is a prerequisite for safely reaching your destination. Angela, however, goes far beyond rational concern for her safety. Essentially, Angela is telling herself: 'Wouldn't it be *awful* if I died before my time!' Granted, it would be most unfortunate if Angela died before she had lived some three score and ten years, which is about the *average* life expectancy nowadays. But why would it be *awful*? Admittedly, death is the worst thing that happens to most of us. But where is the awfulness in not reaching that average of seventy years? Many, many people born on this planet die in their infancy; many more die before they reach young adulthood. And, of course, countless millions die long before they reach seventy from a multitude of causes. Some extremely unfortunate individuals suffer such a high degree of unremitting pain that they practically beg for death to release them from their agony. A fear of dying 'before your time' is really a demand for certainty. In effect, Angela is demanding that God or the universe guarantee her a long life. Where is the evidence that *anyone* is guaranteed *anything* in life? There does not seem to be any certainty in the universe, except the fact that you will *eventually* die. But there is no way of knowing exactly when, where or how that will happen to you. Demanding that you live for x years when you know that there is no possible way your demand can ever be met is surely nothing more than demanding that life be different than it obviously is. If you cling to such an irrational philosophy, how can you ever be anything other than continually anxious? For if you believe you *must* achieve a certain goal and there is no certainty that you will achieve it, you will tend to worry constantly about the possibility of *not* getting what you think you *must* get.

Furthermore, worrying about dying at a young age will certainly not help you to live, or live happily. Quite the contrary! There is good medical evidence that worry itself will help bring on various pathological conditions, such as ulcers or high blood pressure, that might lead to your dying sooner that you otherwise might. In any case you will hardly enjoy whatever life you do have if you keep worrying about when it is going to come to an end.

Angela is also telling herself: 'I *can't stand* the thought of being prevented from having what I've worked for and deserve.' Here again we have an example of LFT. It would certainly be nice if we always got what we considered we deserved. But is there some law in the universe which says we *must* get what we deserve? As far as we can tell, the universe doesn't care one iota whether human beings get what they think they deserve. 'I can't stand the uncertainty of not knowing what is going to happen to me' is a godlike command that life must be easy for me and give me what I want. Can you see that this is just another demand for certainty? The world functions the way it does; whatever happens, happens; there is no evidence that some power is working to give us what we deserve. If you look around you, it is quite easy to believe that the dice are loaded against us getting what we believe we deserve!

And finally, Angela is demanding: 'I *must* have at least twenty years' more life to do what I want, or else life isn't really worth living.' Well, there is no reason, of course, why you should or must live a long and happy life. If there were some law of the universe which said we must live long and happily, then obviously we would. It may well be unfair if you die young and someone else lives until the age of 93. But who said that things *must* be fair? Ask yourself: '*Why* do I *have to* live a long and fairly painless life?' Where is it written that you *have to* do *anything*, for that matter?

By persisting along these lines we would gradually help Angela to see that her highly exaggerated fears and demands are untenable. As she begins to give up her demanding, her '*musturbation*', Angela would probably end up with a different way of looking at things: 'There is no evidence that I *must* not die at an early age. Even if I avoid travelling on motorways and thereby eliminate the possibility of death from that direction, there are numerous other ways in which I might die over which I have little or no control. If I do find myself in that unfortunate situation, then I do! Tough luck! It surely will be very unfortunate if I do not live till I'm in my seventies, but I can't prove it would be terrible if I die before my time and I definitely can stand the thought of it. Worse things have befallen other people and I would be wise to concentrate upon making the most of the time I do have to live instead of wasting it in senseless worry over when my own death will occur. There is no reason why I have to live a long and happy life with my family, though it certainly will be fortunate if I do.'

Here we are making the point that to express a strong desire or preference to achieve your goals in life is fine and healthy: whereas to demand or dictate that life *must* accord you your wishes is both irrational and anxiety-provoking. Coming to these new, rational conclusions, Angela will tend to lose her feelings of panic at the thought of an early demise and replace them with appropriate concern. We would try to help Angela to see that her demand for certainty that her life must go as she wants it is the root cause of her exaggerated fear of motorways, rather than any evidence that motorways are excessively dangerous in themselves, or even more dangerous than other modes of travel. In addition to helping Angela acquire a more realistic outlook on life, we would try to encourage her to *act* against her unrealistic fears of driving on motorways. At first, she would be encouraged to take short journeys on motorways, driving herself a few miles at a time until she came to see that there was nothing exceptionally fearful about doing so. If she still felt over-anxious on entering the motorway, we would try to get her to feel more relaxed by teaching her simple relaxation techniques and 'anti-awfulizing' statements (such as, 'If I do find myself in that unfortunate situation, then I do! Tough luck! I can't prove it would be terrible if I die before my time and I can stand it if it happens'), which she could memorize and repeat to herself when required. As Angela felt less upset, she could then concentrate upon the *process* of driving and use her skill and knowledge to drive to the best of her ability, rather than allow herself to dwell upon the dangers she might encounter and drive with *too* much vigilance, and *too* much caution – which can cause as many problems as not being careful enough.

Once Angela was able to drive short distances on the motorway without feeling too anxious in the process, we would step up her assignments by getting her to drive longer and longer distances until she felt comfortable about driving. Eventually, if she were able to make the journey to her family entirely by motorway and still felt relatively free of anxiety, we would consider that Angela had largely overcome her anxiety problem. She might still feel traces of anxiety from time to time, but that would be acceptable. As long as she felt only a little fear she would still be in control. We would not want her to have no fear at all about driving on motorways, because that would encourage a blasé, over-confident approach which might well bring about the very disaster Angela had previously been so terrified of.

Overcoming the vicious circle of anxiety

We mentioned earlier the vicious circle of anxiety; now let us explain this in greater detail. Once you have experienced anxiety 'for no good reason', you then bring an anxious attitude to the prospect of becoming anxious. You think something like, 'Wouldn't it be terrible if I got anxious.' Thinking in this way actually leads to anxiety. You then notice your anxiety and think something like, 'This is terrible, I'm getting anxious.' This leads to increased anxiety which triggers a further thought like, 'Oh, I'm losing control. What if I faint (or panic, or have a heart attack, or act crazily)? Wouldn't that be terrible!' Anxiety is again heightened, which leads to more anxious 'thinking' and so on. Now this pattern occurs incredibly quickly and you probably are only aware of a building sense of panic.

In addition, you may be one of a large number of people who 'overbreathe' when you become anxious. This means that you take in too much oxygen and feel, paradoxically, that you need to breathe in more air, whereas you actually need less. 'Overbreathing' leads to such sensations as faintness, giddiness and heart palpitations. Without knowing this, you may consider that these sensations are evidence that there really is something wrong with you. This thought leads to more anxiety and the vicious circle continues.

Without the presence of the anxious attitude of 'Wouldn't it be terrible', panic would probably not occur even if you tend to overbreathe, so it is this anxious attitude that you need to identify and change if the seeds of a solution to the problem are to be sown. However, very few people understand this. Hence, what you may have done is avoid situations where you fear you might be anxious. If you don't avoid these situations you may continue to face the anxiety-provoking situation by using a number of common techniques which are designed to distract yourself from your anxiety (relaxation, counting to ten, drinking, etc.). These can be helpful in the short term but more often do not solve the problem – indeed, the use of alcohol to quell anxiety is positively hazardous.

Develop an anti-anxiety attitude

What can be done? First, distinguish between the descriptions 'uncomfortable' and 'terrible'. 'Terrible' probably means to you literally the end of the world. Anxiety is not the end of the world. It is uncomfortable, very uncomfortable at times, but it is not terrible unless you define it as such. If you do define anxiety as terrible then you will take another trip around your vicious circle. So first, if you get anxious, you have to show yourself that anxiety is uncomfortable, bad, inconvenient but that it is not dangerous and it is not the end of the world.

Second, show yourself this in the situation you have tended to shy away from. This sounds simple, and it is; *but it is not easy*! Remember this distinction, it is an important one. You have trained yourself to think that anxiety is terrible and your body reacts to this definition. It is going to take some time for you to retrain yourself to think that anxiety, while most uncomfortable, is not terrible. And it will take longer for your body to react to your new definition.

Third, we have found the following principle, which we developed some years ago, to be very useful. We call it 'challenging but not overwhelming'. By this we mean that if you believe that a situation would be overwhelming for you, then it is perhaps better not to face it yet. But it would be a mistake to go very gradually and only do things that you can do comfortably. Overcoming anxiety means tolerating discomfort, so it is important to face and not shy away from feeling uncomfortable. So choose to start with an experience you will find a challenge. If you don't succeed with this, remember that that is unfortunate, not terrible. Keep applying this principle of challenging but not overwhelming. Choose a challenging situation, face it and practise adopting the attitude of 'anxiety is most uncomfortable, but not terrible' while you are facing it. If you fear you might panic, remember that panic (or a 'ten' as sufferers sometimes call it) lasts only for a very short time even though it seems endless at the time. So use the same attitude to panic: 'If I panic, I panic; that's very unfortunate, but not terrible.'

Lose your fear of ridicule

Now we want to cover one important feature which a large number of our clients have said is also involved in this circle. If you fear that you may act stupidly or crazily and will attract other people's scornful attention as a result, we can tell you that this is unlikely to happen. To convince yourself of this, imagine that it will happen and practise another anti-anxiety attitude. Now if you have this fear it is likely that you believe that if you act stupidly or crazily then this proves you are worthless (useless, stupid, a fool, or whatever word you personally use to condemn yourself). But the problem is not that other people scorn you. It is your agreement with their reaction that is the problem. You think: 'If they think I'm stupid, they're right – I am.' So, once again, it is your attitude towards yourself that is the problem here. Now what you need to ask yourself is this: 'Am I worthless or useless for acting this way, or am I a fallible human being (and equal to others) with a problem?' We hope you realize that you are the latter. If a good friend acted stupidly in public would you condemn him, or would you adopt a compassionate attitude of acceptance towards him? Most probably you would accept him. But he is human like you. So you can practise this accepting attitude towards yourself: 'If I act stupidly that would be bad, but I'm a fallible human being with a problem.' Our clients report that this attitude helps them realize, first, that they are not likely to act stupidly or crazily; second, even if they did act stupidly, other people probably would not condemn them; and third, even if other people did condemn them this would not be the end of the world.

Gain control of your breathing

If you do tend to overbreathe it is important that you gain control of your breathing. This requires a lot of practice and is best done initially under the supervision of a knowledgeable person such as a clinical or counselling psychologist. Controlled breathing involves taking smooth, slow, regular and fairly shallow (not deep!) breaths. Breathe in through your nose and out through your mouth in regular (in-out) cycles. Twelve such cycles per minute is often helpful, but find your own comfortable breathing rhythm. These cycles regulate the amount of oxygen you take in so that you do not experience the tingling, fainting, giddy sensations and the palpitations which are associated with overbreathing.

Applying these anti-anxiety attitudes and techniques like controlled breathing does unfortunately require lots of practice but we have seen many of our clients make steady progress (though setbacks do occur and are to be expected) and we predict if you closely follow these guidelines you will also learn to escape from your own vicious circle of anxiety.

The importance of taking action

While we have emphasized the process of challenging and disputing those irrational beliefs which underlie emotional disturbance, and replacing them with more factual, reality-based ideas, we also wish to stress the importance of *acting* against your previously exaggerated fears. It is all very well to surrender your faulty notions and demands and replace them with a saner philosophy of living. But until you actually *do* what you were previously too fearful to do, your newly acquired attitudes will only be 'skin deep'. Action counterattacks anxiety-producing ideas as few other methods do. It is one of the most effective ways of changing your irrational beliefs available. Not that there is any magic in it; by itself it might not even work sometimes. You can force yourself to drive on some really busy road, for example, and become more and more afraid with every trip you make. But if you take a double-barrelled approach to overcoming your needless fears, if you challenge and question the nonsensical assumptions you make and which lead you to become anxious, *while* acting against your anxieties, you will help yourself to overcome these anxieties. Not that it will be easy! All this may sound simple, but it isn't easy. Deeply rooted anxieties don't just melt away. You have to work, and work hard to get rid of them. When you find it difficult to get going, or continue to avoid doing what you know you had better do, you can use a number of self-management procedures to help yourself.

Action is one of the best antidotes against anxiety. This is true because over-concern is itself a great inhibitor of many human activities. It induces you *not* to do such things as undertaking a surgical operation when the best medical advice strongly indicates it would be in your best interest. It induces you *not* to do such things as flying (if you have a fear of flying), or driving on a busy motorway, as was the case with Angela. Over-concern helps you to *imagine* that these things are much more fearsome than they actually are. If Angela does not drive on motorways, she can easily keep convincing herself that motorway driving is unpleasant, nerve-wracking and dangerous. At the intellectual level, she may not agree that her fears are over-exaggerated and irrational, but so long as she refrains from driving she will still find the idea of motorway driving anxiety-provoking. But if Angela forces herself to drive she will have a difficult time maintaining her irrational fears. This, then, is why we attach importance to what we call 'homework assignments'. We know very well that people can debate with themselves, dilly-dally and avoid doing things forever. But once they are given a concrete homework assignment to do the things they feel afraid to do, and once they force themselves to carry out their assignment, they conquer some of their deepest-seated anxieties quite quickly.

Some valuable self-management techniques

There are various techniques you can employ to help you start doing something you know you had better do but are still afraid of doing. We will be describing several techniques you can employ to help yourself overcome various emotional problems as you read through this book. Here, for example, is one way of motivating yourself to take some action, known as the *principle of reinforcement*. The psychologist, David Premack, discovered that when an individual is reinforced (rewarded) for carrying out some action previously found difficult, that action tends to become easier, and, after a while, semi-automatic, provided the reward or reinforcement is something the individual finds easy and pleasurable. For example, if you keep putting off going to the dentist, or you are finding great difficulty in getting down to writing that special report for your boss, you can single out something you enjoy doing and that you do easily, such as having a drink with your friends, or reading an interesting book – and only allow yourself to do that enjoyable thing *after* you have kept your dental appointment, or spent at least a couple of hours on writing your report. In this way, you reward yourself *as a consequence* of carrying out the unpleasant or difficult task; if you do this often enough, the chances are the set task will become so easy and semi-automatic that you may ultimately not need any reward to do it.

You can use the same approach with anything you want to do but are still stopping yourself from attempting. Think of several things you like to do and can do easily. Using this method, you refrain from reading that great book, or going skiing, or spending a weekend with your boyfriend or girlfriend *until* you have first performed the task you set yourself. Keep persisting with carrying out your homework assignments! Make it difficult for yourself to back down by committing yourself in advance. Tell your boss you are coming round to his office personally with your completed report at a certain time on a certain date. In order to get out of that, you would have to go to the trouble of notifying your boss and making excuses you may not care to make.

If positive reinforcement doesn't get you moving, try applying a penalty! Make a commitment to carrying out some action you want to perform and inform a friend of your decision. Tell your friend to monitor you, and promise that if you fail to carry out your assignment, you will donate a sum of money to some political or religious cause you heartily detest. Make the sum of money large enough to hurt if you were to lose it. Then give the money to your friend to hold for you. If you fail to carry out your assignment, you'll be surprised how highly motivated you will have become the next time you set out to do it!

Finally, accept the possibility – or rather, the probability – that from time to time you will fail to carry out an assignment, and revert, albeit temporarily, to your old anxiety-creating moods. If and when you do, this does not mean that you have to criticize yourself savagely. If you tell yourself that you are a dead loss because you experience once again an attack of anxiety, you will become convinced that a 'dumbo' like you could not *possibly* do any better; and then you will feel more anxious and self-deprecating than ever. Remember, anxiety is only one of the results of self-abasement. You would do much better to convince yourself that, 'It's in my own best interests to carry out this assignment because otherwise it's most unlikely that I will ever get over my silly fear. But I'm not a worthless person if I don't carry out the assignment and I can lead a happy existence even if I never do the assignment. The point is, I can lead a decidedly *happier* life if I do follow through on the assignment; and since I see no real reason why I cannot act so as to

27

enhance my living, I'd jolly well better get cracking. Let's have no more nonsense: I'm going to do this assignment if it's the last thing I do!'

Uproot your anxiety

Regardless of the particular kind of anxiety you may be experiencing – whether it's a 'social anxiety' intimately related to an underlying or overt dread of making public mistakes, of losing someone's love, of antagonising other people, or 'discomfort anxiety' stemming from a demand for certainty that life be predictable and without too many hassles – realize that you are creating your own anxiety through your *shoulds, oughts,* or *musts.* Resolutely track down the major absolutistic generalizations you make which create your needless anxieties, and if you then analyse these generalizations logically to see how they arose and to what conclusions they lead, you will invariably find, first that they are definitional; second, that they impede happy living and are impractical as a means of achieving it; and third, that they lead to unwarranted conclusions. Doing this analysis rigorously will help you give them up. If you consistently keep working at this kind of questioning, you can uproot any conceivable superstition. For that is what negative assumptions about yourself and the world essentially are – groundless superstitions. Remember, any time you demand certainty, you set yourself up for strong feelings of anxiety. The phrase 'Wouldn't it be awful if . . .' is nothing but such a demand. What, then, is the truly elegant solution to this problem? Obviously: give up being so demanding and return to healthy desiring and preferring. Stop escalating your wishes and desires into absolute imperatives! By all means strongly desire and actively work to improve the quality of your life and the social environment in which you live, but do not grandiosely *dictate* that life be otherwise than it indubitably is. Acknowledge that nothing can ever be more than 100 per cent bad, obnoxious, inconvenient or frustrating, and that there is no reason why pains and displeasures *should not* or *must not* exist. Accept once and for all that you *do* live in a world of probability and chance; that almost anything may happen to you, and that you can still be a happy human being in spite of this, or even because of it. Some degree of chance can add variety, interest and excitement to your life. Once you fully convince yourself that certainty is just about impossible to have, and that you may die at any moment (although you probably won't), you can cast off your anxiety, relax and *live.*

Life is for living!

Accept the fact that human existence works according to the laws of probability and chance, and that a certain amount of risk-taking or adventure is what life is really about. Admittedly, risk-taking has its disadvantages; if you are an inveterate gambler, or spend a great deal of your time rock-climbing or participating in motor-racing, you will frequently fail and possibly do yourself harm. But true living does consist, as we have noted, of taking risks. We caution you against being foolhardy and taking risks where the odds are stacked heavily against you. Instead, try for goals that you are not sure you can achieve; look for novelties you are not sure you will enjoy; experimentally determine what it is that you really like and dislike and want to do with your life. There are no purposes to life except those you yourself ascribe to it. If you allow yourself to become terribly worried about death or anything else, inevitably you will take only minimal risks – and usually reap only minimal rewards. The old proverb, 'Nothing ventured, nothing gained', contains a great deal of truth. If you want to live fully, to be *really* alive, you'd better stop worrying about dying or anything else, and do exactly that – take a few risks, and *let* yourself live!

In sum, if you want to conquer your anxieties about death, losing love or about anything else, check your assumptions. Look for your 'shoulds', 'oughts' and 'musts'; observe how you keep saying to yourself, on one level or another, 'Wouldn't it be terrible if . . . ' Then examine these assumptions, logically show yourself how they cannot stand up to critical examination, scientifically question your 'shoulds', 'oughts' and 'musts', and vigorously challenge every 'Wouldn't it be terrible if . . . ' If you change your superstitious thinking, you will change your anxiety reactions to such thinking. Right, go ahead and think! And don't forget that you can substantially reinforce your changed thinking by effective action techniques.

Conclusion

The worst thing about almost any 'disaster' is your exaggerated *belief* in its horror rather than anything intrinsically terrible about it. Life holds innumerable frustrations for all of us; but terrors, horrors, are almost entirely figments of our imagination. Don't be ashamed about still-existing anxieties, no matter how ridiculous they may seem. Admit that you are needlessly fearful and forthrightly tackle your silly worries using the advice and techniques we have outlined in this chapter. But don't waste a minute berating yourself for being, for the moment, unduly afraid. You have much better things to do with your time! And remember, as a mortal human being you have your limitations. You will probably never *completely* overcome all groundless fears and anxieties; life is an unceasing battle against irrational worries because we not only *learn* to worry, we also have an innate propensity to do so. But if you fight this battle intelligently and unremittingly, you can *almost* always be free from most of your needless concerns. What more can you ask of a good life?

SUMMARY POINTS FOR CHAPTER 2

(1) Distinguish fear from anxiety. Fear of actual or potential life-threatening situations is a healthy reaction and tends to be life-preserving. Anxiety is over-concern about the possibility of some 'dreaded' future occurrence which would publicly reveal some personal weakness and thereby imply a loss of self-worth. Anxiety can also follow from the philosophy that life must be easy and comfortable and that it would be awful if it were not.

(2) Feelings of anxiety can be traced back to some variation of the irrational belief 'Wouldn't it be awful if . . .' followed by 'I couldn't stand it if such-and-such were to happen'.

(3) Use the A-B-C model to ferret out the irrational ideas with which you create your anxiety and act effectively against your irrational fears.

(4) Learn to control your breathing if you find yourself tending to overbreathe during an anxiety attack. Fear of becoming anxious may bring on such an attack. You can lower your anxiety level by forcing yourself to face situations which you find uncomfortable but can tolerate without feeling panic.

(5) Use one or more of the self-management techniques given to help you get started whenever you experience difficulty in carrying out actions designed to counterattack your anxiety-creating thoughts.

(6) Anxiety inhibits you from achieving your individual potential for living life to the fullest extent your circumstances allow. Avoid unduly hazardous risks if you will, but realize that living inherently involves risk and that a life lived without risk would hardly be worth living.

3

Depression

Depression is a common emotional disturbance and can be quite debilitating. People tend to see depression as an illness which needs to be treated as such, whereas worrying about the state of the world, or their health, is seen as perfectly normal. As for getting furious with folk who do things they 'shouldn't' do – that is seen as a problem only when it leads to homicide or physical violence. We will be showing you in Chapter 5 that anger, too, usually leads to unfortunate results for yourself as well as for other people. We mention anxiety and anger here because they are both closely linked to depression. All three stem from some combination of irrational ideas which people impose upon themselves and others, and which lead to unfortunate results, emotionally and physically. This is indeed fortunate, because if your depression comes about as a result of the way you talk to yourself about what happens to you, rather than because of some external factor in the world, like a virus or bacterium over which you have no control, then it logically follows that by changing your thinking, you may change the emotional consequences of your thinking.

Now we're going to come straight to the point. We are going to show you how people make themselves depressed, how they keep their depression going, and how they can prevent themselves from becoming depressed in the future. If you follow our advice and work at applying it, you can learn how to deal with virtually any psychologically-based depression* which may afflict you, and get over the pain of it for the rest of your life. And all this without having to swallow a single anti-depressant pill!

However, a word of caution! Unlike the anti-depressant pill your doctor may prescribe, we are not about to offer you a 'quick fix' for your depression. While these pills you swallow may help you *feel* better temporarily, they are unlikely to help you to *get* better, because they do not get to the psychological core of the depression. We are not offering palliative solutions to depression, or indeed to any other kind of emotional upset. What we aim to achieve is to teach you how depression is caused, and what you can do to overcome it using the principles and techniques of Rational-Emotive Therapy (RET), which

---

*Some types of depression are biologically-based, and we recommend that you see your doctor for advice about this subject before applying our suggestions, if you cannot readily find any psychological reasons for your depression.

have proved workable and successful in numerous instances of individuals suffering from depression.

Some people may find it more difficult than others to overcome depressive episodes. There is evidence that the biochemical balance in the body may render some people more prone to experience depressed moods than other people. Be that as it may, the fact of being susceptible to the onset of depression does not mean that depression will necessarily occur. Modern health research workers now subscribe to the view that the state of our health – and our susceptibility to various illnesses – is a function of several aspects of our lifestyle, including the fitness of our immune response as well as the state of our mind. So, don't let yourself get downhearted! The methods we will teach you in this book to overcome your emotional upsets will stand you in good stead, regardless of your individual circumstances. Should you be so unfortunate as to experience a really severe depression which virtually incapacitates you, a spell in hospital with some medication may be necessary before you can begin to think clearly enough to tackle the problem. For example, if you ran down and killed a child while driving your car, you might well feel so shattered with guilt and remorse, that you would be quite incapable of doing anything for a while. It would clearly be unrealistic to counsel you while you were in a state of shock and under sedation. But once the initial shock had subsided enough to permit you to start to put your life together again, your depression could be tackled using the methods we are about to outline.

Three causes of depression

We agree with Dr Paul Hauck, a noted American psychologist, who has argued that there are basically three routes through which you can become depressed: self-denigration; self-pity; and other-pity.* Though we will consider each separately, you should bear in mind that they are not mutually exclusive – a person can become depressed through both self-denigration and self-pity, for example – and that there is considerable overlap between the irrational beliefs underlying them.

Self-denigration

People who denigrate or despise themselves, frequently do so when they fail to live up to their standards and when they demand that they must not fail. This may happen at work, or it may occur in some personal relationship. In each case, the self-depreciation which may

*Dr Paul Hauck, *Depression* (Sheldon Press, 1974); *How To Be Your Own Best Friend* (Sheldon Press, 1988), also the writer of our Foreword

follow the failure to perform well, or even outstandingly, leads to depression. Why so? Well, let's take a closer look at what it means to live up to one's standards. There's nothing inherently wrong in setting yourself certain standards in your work, as well as in your personal life. In fact, certain standards or levels of attainment are generally expected in business, in the professions, in the field of art, and so on. As an individual, you have certain main goals and purposes in life, and it will usually be in your interest to achieve them through acquiring the requisite degrees of competence or expertise your particular field expects of you. To strive for a high level of performance in the pursuit of your personal and professional goals is fine; to succeed in achieving your goals is usually personally satisfying and rewarding in material and other ways.

Now, if you *only* desire or strongly prefer something (such as living up to certain standards in your vocation and winning the approval or love of those people whom you choose to make important to you), you would virtually never seriously upset yourself about the possibility of not fulfilling your desire. For you would be saying to yourself: 'I am trying to reach a high standard in carrying out this assignment because I see it is important to me to do so, and to win so-and-so's approval – but if I fail, I fail! It isn't the end of the world. Now, let me see where I slipped up, and if I can eliminate my errors I may be able to do well the next time and win so-and-so's approval later; and if I never succeed with this particular job and win her approval, that's really tough! And that's it–too bad!' How do you think you would feel if you held these kinds of beliefs about your failure? Well, you would feel sorry, probably very disappointed and very sad – but *not* depressed or suicidal!

Alas! Because we are all too human, we find it easy to go beyond strongly *desiring* to achieve our standards and win approval from people who are important to us. Thus, in terms of our A-B-C model of emotional disturbance, at point A you are trying to achieve certain standards in some task or activity; you might, for example, be engaged in preparing a special report for your board competition, or trying hard to be a competent student. But you fail to reach your desired level of performance and you are criticized and rejected by some significant person whose approval you've attached great importance to winning. At point B, as we have shown, your *rational* beliefs about what has happened to you, would be of the order of: 'I would like to have done well and achieved the level of performance I was aiming to achieve, and to have won the approval of someone I respect; but I didn't, and that is annoying. I am a person who failed to reach the standards I set for myself. Too bad!' Naturally, at point C (the emotional consequence), you would feel regretful and frustrated.

At point B, however, you also cling to a much stronger set of *irrational* beliefs: 'I *must* do well at these projects of mine and win the approval of people who are important to me. And since I failed to do what I *must* do, it's *awful*! I can't *stand* it! I'm just no good at all for acting so ineptly!' You then also, at point C, feel anxious and depressed. As we have been pointing out in this, and in previous chapters, what we generally label emotional difficulties – feelings of severe anxiety, depression, worthlessness – almost invariably stem from people's tendency to escalate strong, legitimate desires and preferences into overwhelming and illegitimate demands, commands and *musts*. The solution, then, to ridding yourself of any psychologically-based depression is to uproot your negative, self-defeating philosophies which created it in the first place and help sustain it in the second place. To do that, you move on to point D – D stands for *disputing*

How to dispute your self-denigrating beliefs When we dispute a belief or conviction, we use the scientific method. That is to say, we ask questions designed to establish whether the belief or conviction is based on solid fact and whether it can be logically upheld. For example, we would ask: 'Does this belief or theory offer us the best explanation of the observed facts? Show us the data on which it is based.' Using this method we would dispute the irrational beliefs which create and sustain your depression as follows.

First, where is the evidence that you *must* do well at your projects and win the approval of certain people? Well, there seems to be no evidence for either of these *musts*! If there was some law of the universe which said that you *must* do well and win the approval of certain people, things would be arranged such that you could not fail to do just that. Since, however, you quite obviously did not do what you thought you *must* do, you may legitimately suspect that no such law exists. Of course, it would have been highly desirable if you had done well and lived up to your standards and won favour from people whose approval you valued. But it does not follow that because you strongly want something, you *must* be granted it! That may be *your* law, but there is no evidence so far that the universe intends to obey it!

Second, in what way is it *awful* when you don't live up to your standards and gain the support of people who mean a lot to you? It is certainly unfortunate when you perform poorly and alienate or antagonize people who matter to you – because then you are not getting what you wanted. But when you call something awful, or terrible, you really mean that it is more than just plain bad. Isn't that quite an exaggeration? When you tell yourself that it is *awful* that you failed and

34

were rejected, you really mean that your failure is not only bad, but is in some respects *totally*, or 100 per cent bad. Isn't that more than just a little unlikely? If it were really 100 per cent bad that you failed, it follows that no good whatsoever could ever come of it. In fact, a considerable amount of good could come from your failing to do well this time; you could learn from your mistakes and try to do better next time. If certain people you respect rejected you this time, you could accept it as a challenge to win their approval another time. You could, alternatively, get to know others who are more likely to approve of you; or, just as importantly, learn to accept yourself in spite of the fact that certain important people do not like you. It may be 80 or 90 per cent bad if you fail and get rejected, but it can hardly be 100 per cent. Moreover, when a thing is 100 per cent bad, it is as bad as it can possibly be. If it really were 100 per cent bad to fail in some task and be rejected by some person whose approval you wanted, this would mean that you could have no happiness whatsoever for the rest of your life. Isn't that most unlikely – that failing and being rejected this time will deprive you of all happiness for all time?

Third, where is the evidence to support your contention that you *can't stand* failing to live up to your standards and being rejected for failing? There is none! When we say we can't stand something, we are really misusing language. What we mean is, we *won't* stand something – a very different thing! For if we really could not stand a thing, we would literally collapse or come apart at the seams and disintegrate. If, in fact, you could not *bear* to fail at important tasks or win the approval of important people, you wouldn't be able to do anything else; you would have to fail at everything you ever attempted. Obviously, that is untrue. You could do similar tasks and sometimes succeed, and the more you kept trying the more likely you would be to succeed in your enterprises, including the gaining of others' esteem. Yes, you most decidedly *can* stand what you don't like. You *can* stand falling down on some important job or occupation and losing or failing to get the love or approval you seek. You'll never enjoy failure and rejection, but you can gracefully lump it; and provided you don't make a great song and dance about it, but instead calmly and earnestly try to do better next time, you have a good chance of succeeding later and winning some people's approval.

Finally, in what way are you no good for failing to live up to your standards and being disapproved of? In no way can you legitimately label yourself as no good regardless of how many times you perform badly and fail to win the acceptance or approval of significant people in your life. There are several reasons why you cannot legitimately rate yourself in terms of your behaviour. First, your acts, deeds and performances are only aspects of you; they are never the whole of you, never your totality. What we call the *self* is an ongoing, ever-changing process. During your lifetime, you will perform literally millions of actions, some good, some bad; some will win you approval, some will result in censure. You may do a fine job today, and earn everyone's plaudits; tomorrow, you may mess up some project and be derided by your associates as incompetent. Since you consist of innumerable actions, all of which change from day to day, how can you equal any of these actions? You have a past, a present and a future. No matter how poorly you may have done certain things in the past, how could you ever justifiably conclude that you'll *never* be able to do well at these things in a global, once-and-for-all manner? Essentially, what we are saying here is that human worth and worthlessness are definitions which are vague, mystical and unrelatable to reality. To rate someone's *personhood* or *self* is akin to rating his *soul*. How can that be done? Whenever you denigrate yourself for failing to live up to your standards, you are demeaning your *self*, your *essence*, for your unsuccessful deeds.

A second consideration is that if you were a rotten or no-good person, you would consist of some soul or essence that was completely rotten. That is obviously an unprovable proposition. It would mean that you could *only* and *always* do rotten things. This, again, is unprovable, as is also the conclusion to be drawn from it, namely, that because of your rotten acts you don't deserve any good results now, or at any time in the future, no matter how hard you try, and that you are a thoroughly damnable person who deserves to suffer for the rest of your life.

And third, if you see yourself as a rotten or no-good person for having performed badly, how will that view of yourself help you to correct your bad behaviour and do better in the future? If you think about it, you'll see that it won't! The more you view yourself as a no-good *person* who is virtually doomed to behave badly, now and in the future, the more that view will handicap you in your efforts to improve. Your negative view of yourself will become a self-fulfilling prophecy and you will use your continued failures as 'proof' of your worthlessness in the first place. A far more sensible view is to consider yourself as neither good nor bad as a *person*, but as a *fallible* human being who does unfortunate acts but who also has the power to act better in the future. Adopting this view of yourself will help you to perform more successfully, to live up to your standards more frequently and to win greater approval from other people. Don't you think that this view would be more practical and helpful to you than the self-deprecating one of seeing yourself as a worthless individual?

Acquire a self-accepting philosophy If you persist in disputing your irrational and self-denigrating beliefs along the lines we have shown you in the above examples, you will wind up with a new outlook, a new set of philosophical, emotional and behavioural effects, which we call point E. It takes time and effort on your part to get there; but if you actively look for and dispute your irrational beliefs and self-belittling notions you will eventually acquire the ability to react sensibly to life's disappointments rather than depress yourself about them. When, for instance, you do poorly on some project and incur the disapproval of certain people, you will conclude at point E: 'Yes, unquestionably I blew that particular job and brought on my head disapproval from some important people. And since I am a fallible, error-prone human, I will probably continue to slip up from time to time and do myself less than justice; I know I *can* do better, but because neither I nor anyone else is perfect, I can live with the probability that today I might do well, while tomorrow I might do badly. That is too bad, and distinctly unfortunate for me in various ways. But it isn't the end of the world. I can still be fairly happy in spite of my failing and in spite of losing the love or approval of many of those I would like to have impressed with my abilities. Again, too bad! If that's the way it is, that's the way it is. I can continue to live and enjoy myself by accepting reality and by trying to do a little better and win somewhat more approval in future. Realistically, that is all I am able to do.' With that philosophy and outlook, you can feel sorry and regretful when you fail at important tasks, rather than anxious and depressed; and you will then find you have given yourself leeway to act and behave more efficiently and more self-helpfully in the future so that you make fewer mistakes and gain more (though never complete) approval from those people you prefer to be associated with.

Self-pity

Depression resulting from self-pity often occurs after some loss, such as the loss of some loved one through death, or the loss of a job. The depressed person is thinking something like: 'Why me? What have I done to deserve this? I'll never be able to get a replacement and be happy again. What a rotten life this is!' Ideas like these, which boil down to 'Life is too hard', 'I can't stand it', 'Poor me, I'll never be able to manage on my own' and 'It will be so uncomfortable, I couldn't live with that situation', are variations of one of the major irrational ideas we introduced in the first chapter, and which may be paraphrased as follows: 'The conditions under which I live must be so arranged that I get practically everything I want comfortably, quickly and easily, and my life absolutely must not be filled with hassles particularly when I've done nothing to deserve them. When it does, I can't bear it and the world becomes a thoroughly rotten place that is not worth living in.' This irrational idea will almost inevitably result in feelings of self-pity and resentment, and these, in turn, may lead to low frustration tolerance and other self-defeating behaviours.

A case of self-pity Take the case of Mary, a 47-year-old audio secretary who is separated from her husband who walked out on her. 'I feel so hurt', says Mary. Dabbing her eyes with a handkerchief, she continues: 'I didn't drive him away. How could he ever think of going with another woman after all I've done for him over the years! It's so terribly unfair of him to treat me like this! When I think of how I've slaved away for him, doing a full-time job and making a comfortable home for him, and then he goes and does a thing like this to me! Is this all I deserve after twenty-one years of marriage?' Let's put this example of self-pitying hurt into the A-B-C framework and see how we could use it to help Mary to get over her depression and deal more effectively with her marital situation.

The A-B-C of self-pity First of all, note that Mary infers from her husband's departure that he has acted in an 'unfair' manner towards her and that she considers herself totally undeserving of such treatment. At point A, Mary's husband walks out on her. This is the activating event. At point C, Mary feels hurt and full of self-pity. This is the emotional consequence. Most people would think that A causes C. Not so! As we have already shown you, if A always caused C, that would mean that every time one marriage partner walked out on the other, the abandoned one would have to feel hurt and self-pity. Some people would, undoubtedly. Others would feel sad, disappointed, or even annoyed. Still others would get out the champagne. The same activating event, A, can be followed by several different emotional and behavioural consequences at C. The reason why different people react in different ways to a given situation or event is, as we have stressed, because of what they *believe* about the event. In our model, point B stands for the person's system of beliefs about what happens to him or her at point A.

So let's look at what Mary is telling herself about the fact of her husband's desertion. Like everyone else, Mary brings her own set of beliefs and evaluations to bear upon the various events at A, the activating events in her life. So, at point B, we would expect to find that Mary holds some fairly specific beliefs about being deserted. We would expect to find that some of her beliefs are quite sensible or rational. We know that Mary does not suffer from brain damage; she is capable of making rational judgements. If she hadn't been capable of discriminating fact from fancy, she probably would not have survived the major part of her forty-seven years. Instead, she would have been looked after in an institution. But Mary has survived and coped quite well with her life. So, just what are Mary's beliefs, her core ideas if you like, about her husband leaving her?

At point B, Mary holds a number of rational beliefs – that is to say, her rational beliefs are supported by facts and are confirmable. One of these is: 'I shall be inconvenienced in many ways as a direct result of my husband leaving me. Things will be difficult for me financially, and my standard of living will be affected. I will probably find myself on my own more often than I care to be.' She is also telling herself: 'I would much prefer it if he hadn't left.' Now, if Mary stayed rigorously with these beliefs, she would feel disappointed at the way her marriage had turned out, and she would feel sad as she recollected some of the good times she and her husband had shared in the past. She might even feel annoyed that her husband had not appreciated her contribution to the marriage and their mutual happiness sufficiently to make him want to stay. By sticking to these rational beliefs – the kind of beliefs Mary would easily put to a woman friend facing a similar situation, Mary would feel sad and displeased, but certainly not hurt and self-pitying.

Unfortunately, Mary's rational observations and beliefs about her situation are overshadowed by a much stronger set of *irrational* observations and beliefs. These are the beliefs which Mary really holds deep down inside her and which create her emotional turmoil. For Mary is telling herself, 'My husband *absolutely should not* have treated me in such an unfair manner' and: 'It's terrible to be treated in this way, particularly since I don't deserve to be. Poor me! And what a rotten, unjust world this is that allows such unfairness to exist! I *absolutely shouldn't* get what I don't deserve.' With beliefs like these, it is little wonder that Mary feels hurt and depressed.

At the same time, Mary's behaviour changed. Before her husband left her, Mary had been active in a number of ways. She had played golf and had been a member of the local arts and crafts group. But as she became more and more sorry for herself, her depression deepened and her social life became non-existent. Mary became inert, and appeared to have lost interest in her friends and previous activities. This withdrawal into oneself is typical behaviour when people make themselves depressed. Another common behavioural reaction to depression occurs when the person starts smoking or drinking, or gets involved in self-defeating activities such as drug-taking, or uncharacteristic sexual activities. You may also observe remarkable switches in the person's more deeply held convictions and tastes. These all serve the purpose of enabling the depressed person temporarily to escape from, and cover up, the pain of depression.

To help her overcome her depression, Mary was shown that it was her irrational beliefs about her husband's desertion that largely created her emotional distress. First, we helped Mary to see that her belief that her husband had unfairly treated her, and that he had acted inconsiderately in walking out on her in the way that he did, was essentially an inference on her part. It may have been true, of course, but without knowing more about the husband's motives, we could not be sure. We know for a fact that some husbands walk out on their wives for reasons which have nothing to do with their wives' own behaviour. Some husbands are so emotionally disturbed, that they have difficulty in getting along with *anyone*, let alone their long-suffering wives! It is important to remember that we all make attributions; we impute motives and intentions to other people to help us understand why they act as they do. We generally perceive the facts of a situation accurately enough, but our interpretations of the meaning behind other people's actions are often wide of the mark. Normally this doesn't matter too much since all that has transpired is that we have misunderstood the real reasons behind some other person's behaviour. However, if we *act* on the basis of an incorrect understanding of the other person's motives, the consequences can be rather unfortunate. One of these consequences is that we can give ourselves a needless pain in the gut whenever we construe some other person's behaviour as deliberately unfair or hostile to us. So, a piece of advice: check your attributions! Do not cavalierly assume that whenever someone acts towards you in a manner which you construe as unfair or unethical, it means they are deliberately trying to do you in. They *may* be, but it is quite possible that they are merely acting out of stupidity or ignorance.

Whether or not Mary's husband acted towards her in an uncaring manner, she thought that he did and considered herself undeserving of such treatment: 'He should not have left me and it's terrible to be treated in such an unfair manner after all I did for him.' Maybe it would have been better for Mary if her husband had stayed in the marriage. In fact, he didn't. But given that *it would have been better* had he stayed, where is the evidence that he *absolutely should not* have left and treated Mary unfairly? There isn't any! The phrase 'it would have been better . . .' makes sense; it expresses a value judgement which has some factual evidence to back it up. But where does 'he absolutely should not . . .' come from? Isn't it a demand or command that somehow the universe must be so ordered that such a thing must not happen? Well, if the universe were so arranged that certain things absolutely must not happen, then they would not happen, because they *could* not happen!

Every time you use the words 'should', 'ought' or 'must' in an absolutistic way, you are grandiosely demanding that the world has to be the way you want it to be, or not to be the way you don't want it to be. These three words, 'should', 'ought' and 'must', have legitimate meaning when used in the conditional sense. For example, it makes sense to say, 'I should take my umbrella if I want to avoid being soaked in this downpour.' But it makes no sense to say, 'You absolutely should have treated me much better than you did.' If you view world events in a rigid, absolute way, you will almost inevitably experience anxiety, depression or anger when you discover that the world does not conform to your dogmatic shoulds, oughts and musts. You will do much better to assume that world events, and especially human affairs, follow the laws of probability.

Continuing in this manner, Mary began to see that her belief that it was 'terrible' to be treated unfairly by her husband (or for that matter, by anybody else), was a gross exaggeration. Admittedly, it can be frustrating and inconvenient when someone treats us unfairly. In Mary's case, she was put to considerable inconvenience and was deprived of several kinds of support through her husband's leaving her. But if we believe that it is 'terrible' when some misfortune occurs, we are not only viewing it as bad, but that it is as bad as bad can be, and therefore could not possibly be worse. How can *anything* be 100 per cent bad? If you cling to the idea that it is 'terrible' to be treated unfairly, and that the world is a rotten place for allowing such 'terrible' things to happen, you may 'logically' conclude that you can never know any happiness again. Is that likely? Could you *never* be happy again? Just suppose that your partner walked out on you, as Mary's did. Is that the worst possible thing that could happen to you? If you think it is, then how would you feel if you *also* broke your leg? Or *also* suffered a stroke and became paralysed from the waist down? Where on your scale of badness from 0 to 100 would losing your partner now be placed? No matter what happens to you, you can always imagine something worse happening to you! Can you see that both of Mary's irrational statements – that her husband should not have treated her so unfairly, and that she should not get what she does not deserve – go far beyond any possibility of logical or scientific verification?

The rational alternative to self-pity The rational alternative to self-pity is to accept that as a human being you have goals in life, and two of your main goals are to survive and be happy. Since we live on a planet peopled by millions of other humans who also have their goals and who try to attain them, there will inevitably be times when conflicts of interests or conflicts over resources may temporarily block us from obtaining what we are seeking, or frustrate the fulfilment of some desire. If you practise seeing the difference between striving for what you want out of life without portraying your desires as absolute necessities, and on the other hand dogmatically demanding that the world be so arranged that you always get what you 'deserve' and do not get what you do not 'deserve', you will tend to enjoy life more, and to live more happily with yourself and other people.

You can do this by looking for your irrational beliefs – your dogmatic shoulds and musts – every time you begin to feel self-pitying. Then, when you find them, eliminate them by challenging and disputing them until you see their absurdity. By understanding and working at uprooting your crazy ideas, you will gain control of your emotional destiny. You may occasionally experience sadness or sorrow, but you will rarely feel self-pityingly depressed again.

Other-pity

Just as you can become depressed through pitying yourself, you can also depress yourself through pitying other people, animals, the loss of a home you've lived in for many years, or even the destruction of a lovely village street as a result of the developers moving in. You can become pitying over almost anything. If the recently widowed lady down the street is evicted from her home, you would feel compassion for her and try to help her to fight for her rights or give practical help in some other appropriate way. But it is easy to go beyond caring and compassion and to slip into depression. The sort of thing you will hear yourself or others saying about the woman's plight is: 'After all she's gone through, how could she deserve what has happened to her now! Isn't it terrible she's suffering so, as she *must* not.'

The irrational idea here is that we should be upset over other people's problems. This does not imply that we can just adopt an uncaring attitude to other people's misfortunes. Each time we see on our TV screens thousands of starving children, or witness the devastation caused to countless others by floods, earthquakes and other natural disasters, we would be uncaring if we did not feel empathy or sensitivity for the sufferings of our fellow man. When we care enough about the misfortunes that happen to others we can take every effective action to try to improve their situation. For example, we can donate money and clothing to relief agencies, or volunteer our help in running them.

However, if you upset yourself over other people's problems, you become less effective in helping them get over their difficulties. It is irrational to say, 'It *shouldn't* happen!' whenever bystanders or passers-by are killed or injured in a bomb blast, for instance. Feeling pity for the victims isn't going to help them much. They want help, practical help, and quickly. You need to keep a cool head in an emergency if you are called to the scene and required to assist the victims in an effective manner. Upsetting yourself over the injuries and distress afflicting those whom you are trying to help will make you less effective than if you refuse to pity the victims and, instead, concentrate your mind and energies in getting these unfortunate people into hospital as quickly as possible.

Remember that whatever happens, happens because the requisite conditions exist for it to happen. If you are concerned about the miserable situation some people are living in, figure out how to do something practical to help them. If you allow yourself to become so upset that you suffer yourself over these others' sufferings, in what way does *your* suffering help lessen *theirs*? If you feel all cut up over the misery you see in the world, how is that going to relieve it? Furthermore, if you were asked to help someone suffering from depression, and you allowed yourself to feel so sympathetic towards the sufferer that you became depressed yourself, you would hardly be showing the sufferer a good undisturbed model to emulate. You would be showing the depressed person by your own upset emotions that he or she had every justification to become upset in the first place; that, faced with his or her situation, you could scarcely avoid becoming depressed yourself! Lavishing sympathy on a depressed person may temporarily help him or her to *feel* better but it will rarely help him or her to *get* better, because reinforcing the person's low tolerance of frustration makes it more difficult for him or her to think and act against self-defeating, strongly entrenched attitudes.

A case of other-pity Take the case of Jane, a 23-year-old university graduate who joined an overseas relief agency to see if she could help to alleviate the appalling conditions under which some poor people in Africa were living. A few months later she returned home feeling acutely depressed. 'It was seeing these starving children', Jane explained. 'What had they done to deserve such a fate?' When she compared her own lot with the miseries she witnessed daily, the burden became so great for Jane that she was unable to eat. Eventually, she was sent home.

'There's no justice in the world!' she cried. 'Life *shouldn't* be like that!' We agreed that there was no justice in this case, and we doubted whether there had ever been a time when everyone received justice. 'But why should there be?' we asked. 'Natural disasters strike without warning. They cause destruction and suffering to some, while other people more fortunate escape. There is no saying who will fall victim

43

and who will escape. If a disaster does not strike us, it will strike someone else. And to the catalogue of natural disasters we add those of our own making. We can do something to reduce or eliminate the latter, but, as yet, there is little we can do about the former. Accept as a fact that reality is ugly for many of us but that bemoaning the fact will do nothing to bring improvement. Why then needlessly upset yourself about the miseries that abound when you could devote your not inconsiderable energies to changing things for the better?' Gradually, Jane came to see that her pity resulted from *over*-concern for the plight of those she worked with. She came to agree that her depression was a thief of both her time and her energy which could have been used to much better advantage. 'Imagine yourself in the place of one of these unfortunate people,' we said. 'Then, ask yourself which would be the more helpful. A day of sympathy and prayer? Or a day's rations? Or even some clean water and antibiotics?'

Let's face it, reality is often far from pretty. Pain, poverty, disease, malnutrition and homelessness are a sad, constant factor in the lives of literally millions of people in this world, each and every day. That's the way it is at present. We can try to make the world – indeed, it would be much better if we could make the world – a healthier, happier place in which to live. And we can do it. But if we wring our hands and deplore the horror of it and the hopelessness of it by believing 'It's *awful*' and 'It *shouldn't* be the way it is', then the chances are it will remain just that way.

Whenever you experience pity for the plight of other people, you are not merely feeling sorry for them. You are straying beyond rational concern into the realm of over-concern, hopelessness and despair. Kindly concern for others is healthy and can be helpful, because it can motivate you into doing something practical to help them overcome their misfortunes. Over-concern is irrational because it causes you anxiety and depression and it is self-defeating and therefore unhelpful to others since these feelings block effective action.

Diversion methods of combating depression

The principle of diversion is one of the best techniques for alleviating the pain of depression, at least temporarily. Your ultimate goal, of course, is to rid yourself of your depression and suicidal thoughts which may accompany it. However, when you are stricken with grief and feeling so deeply depressed that you see no hope for yourself in the future, you need help to interrupt the incessant flow of depression-sustaining thoughts that seem to blot out everything else. If you want to break out of the stranglehold created by those energy-sapping thoughts going round and round in your in your head – such as how awful life has become for you, and how hopeless you now feel that you are ever to know happiness again – some physical activity involving some degree of mental concentration will help you. The human mind is so ordered that it is extremely difficult to concentrate on two quite different things simultaneously. Thus, if you force yourself into several kinds of distracting activity which take your mind off your problem, you will feel a lessening of the pain of depression which will then give your brain a 'breather', so to speak, and thus enable you to begin the process of challenging your suicidal and depression-creating views and replacing them with a rational, more self-helping philosophy.

What sort of techniques can you employ? Well, you can call up or visit friends, or go outside and strike up a conversation with people you encounter in a park. Talk about anything, *except* what you feel depressed about! Or if you normally enjoy music, listen to an interesting piece of music and then try to analyse the performance. Write up notes about it. If you saw some interesting event taking place while you were out, and you are artistically inclined, try drawing or painting a picture of it when you return home. If you can get going on some long-range project, so much the better. The trick is to keep your mind occupied with some project which cannot proceed without your giving it attention. If you persist at it, you will notice one day that you no longer feel quite so down as you did. Avoid routine activities, because since you tend to do these automatically, you leave yourself plenty of time to revert to your depression. Keep yourself involved in some kind of mental effort. A game of chess with a difficult opponent, or something along these lines, will really help you to spring the suicide trap. It may seem hard to get going, but it will be all the harder on you if you don't. You *can* do it. So try! Don't give up until your depressed moods have waned to the point where they no longer are a problem.

At the same time as your persistence in acting against your depression begins to pay off, get cracking on solving the basic problem of depression. None of the diversion techniques we have suggested you use will truly solve the problem of how you became depressed in the first place. All that they will do is to temporarily interrupt your depression-creating philosophy so that it doesn't overwhelm you altogether.

Getting to grips with the core of depression

Remember that, whatever may have contributed to your depressed state, be it the death of some loved person, or the loss of a job, or the break-up of a close relationship, it did not by itself cause you to feel depressed and suicidal. You yourself created your depression through your 'awfulizing' about the particular misfortune which has befallen you. Your aim, therefore, is to uproot the irrational ideas underlying your depression and replace them with rational, realistic ideas using the methods we outlined earlier in the cases of Mary and Jane. Achieving that isn't easy when you see yourself in a 'hopeless' situation, and feel unable to change it for the better. That is why some activity is good for you: action forces you to interrupt the flow of depression-sustaining ideas, such as 'It's *terrible* to lose a job at my age, and I'll *never* be able to get another!' or 'No one cares how I feel, I'm so alone, and life *should not* be so hard for me, especially as I don't *deserve* to suffer like this!' Once you obtain some relief from the pain of depression, you will be in much better shape to focus on your *real* problem: how to replace your irrational demands that 'life must not be too difficult' and that 'unfairness must not exist, or if it does, I can't stand it' with more reality-based views which will help, rather that defeat, your goal of living a reasonably happy life, no matter what hassles and sorrows may still lie ahead of you.

Conclusion

Regardless of how your depression may have come about – through self-denigration, or self-pity or other-pity, or through a combination of them – bear in mind that, in most instances, you created it by your own irrational evaluations of what was happening to you. Whether or not you were prescribed drugs to help you initially overcome your depression, you will find that if you actively and vigorously counter-attack your irrational beliefs using the methods we have taught you, combined with those assignments we gave you to *act* against your depression, you will help yourself to a happier and much less depression-prone existence.

SUMMARY POINTS FOR CHAPTER 3

(1) If you experience severe or chronic depression, and your medical check-up has revealed no organic or physiological factors which could precipitate a depressed state, you may be reasonably sure that the basic cause is psychological.

(2) Depression may arise from a combination of one or two of the following basic emotional states: self-denigration; self-pity; and other-pity. Each of these states comes about because of people's tendency to escalate strong legitimate desires and preferences into overwhelming and illegitimate demands, commands and musts.

(3) The solution to ridding yourself of any psychologically-based depression is to uproot your negative, self-defeating philosophies which created it in the first place and help sustain it in the second place.

(4) To convince yourself that the beliefs underlying your negative philosophies are untenable, you can use the A-B-C model of emotional disturbance to identify and dispute these core irrational beliefs until you really see that they are logically and factually unsupportable. These irrational core beliefs underpinning depression are:

   (a) I *must* achieve and live up to certain standards and win the love or approval of people who are important to me. If I fail to do so, it's awful, because that proves I'm no good and I can't stand that (self-denigration).

   (b) I absolutely *should not* be treated unfairly because I don't deserve to be. Poor me! What a hard, rotten place this world is for allowing such unfairness to exist. I can never be happy again (self-pity).

   (c) I *should* be upset over other people's problems and the poor world conditions under which some unfortunate people live. I can't stand such unfairness and injustice (other-pity).

(5) Determinedly *acting* against your depression in addition to combating the irrational ideas which create and sustain it will help you rid yourself of your depressed feelings more effectively and probably more quickly than either method by itself. A concerted attack upon your depressed state is your best bet for obtaining relief.

(6) If suicide enters your mind, don't toy with the idea. Tell someone how you feel and ask for help in distracting you from your suicidal thoughts by carrying out some suggestions outlined in this chapter. We believe that suicide is rarely justified. Morever, when you are in a depressed state, you are not thinking clearly and rationally and if you go ahead and kill yourself, the chances are you will have made a mistake – a mistake which once made cannot be rectified! Give yourself the benefit of the doubt; after your depression has lifted, you will see life in a different light.

4
Guilt

Anyone who has lived under the shadow of guilt (and virtually all of us have done so at some time or other in our lives), will need no reminding that guilt is one of the most uncomfortable feelings it is possible to have. But what is guilt? And why do people suffering from guilt feel so miserable?

First, let's consider some common definitions of guilt and closely-related concepts. In their *Comprehensive Dictionary of Psychological and Psychoanalytical Terms*, English and English define guilt as the 'Realization that one has violated ethical or moral or religious principles, together with a regretful feeling of lessened personal worth on that account'. In Webster's *New World Dictionary*, 'blame' is defined thus: 'accusation; condemnation; censure, responsibility for a fault or wrong'. Closely related to these definitions is the concept of 'sin' which English and English define as, 'Conduct that violates what the offender believes to be a supernaturally ordained moral code'.

In general terms, therefore, we can say that when an individual feels guilty, part of what that individual believes is that he or she has performed some deed which violates his or her personal code of morals, or rules of behaviour, or that he or she has acted wickedly or wrongly in the eyes of some god or some social value system. However, that is only *part* of what the individual believes or infers. It is what follows those inferences that really creates the feeling of guilt. For in order to *feel* guilty – as distinct from merely inferring that you have acted wickedly or wrongly – you would have to believe: 'I absolutely should not have done what I did, or should have done what I did not. I should be condemned for doing so, or not doing so, and should be punished.' If you did not demand absolutes in your own standard of behaviour, that you be condemned and punished for doing what you shouldn't or for not doing what you should, you would be unlikely to feel guilty. You would, we hope, feel remorse and sorrow, but not guilt, when you commit a wrong, for reasons we will now put before you. Just in passing, however, we hope you are not confusing guilt with shame. Although there is some overlap between shame and guilt in terms of emotional consequences, they are not the same. We shall be dealing with the notion of shame in Chapter 7. Because guilt feelings can be so crippling emotionally, and because a sense of guilt also frequently leads to anxiety, depression and anger, we feel justified in examining this concept of guilt to determine whether a sense of guilt is either inevitable or helpful.

What do we mean by a sense of guilt?

At this point, we anticipate some questions from you before we go any further. 'What's all this about a sense of guilt not being inevitable or helpful? You're surely not implying that if I commit some misdeed, or do someone a wrong, I'm just going to feel quite indifferent about it? Surely anyone is bound to feel guilty when they do something they know is wrong? And if they don't, they jolly well should!' To which we would reply: 'No, we certainly would *not* want you to feel indifferent about your wrongdoing. That is not our intention. By all means acknowledge your responsibility for any misdeed you may commit. Do not evade responsibility for your actions. What we *are* saying – and we hope to convince you presently – is that you need not *feel* guilty, worthless or some kind of blackguard *even* when you do act badly or immorally towards someone.' 'Oh, come now!', we can imagine you exclaiming, as you wonder if we have taken leave of our senses. 'If I do something I know to be wrong, something that violates my deepest principles, surely I'm *bound* to feel guilty and pretty much of a louse?' To which we would respond: 'No, not necessarily!' Please bear with us while we examine how our definition of guilt is formulated.

If you look at it closely, you will see that guilt has three components, expressed in the following statements:

(1) 'I have done the wrong thing and am responsible for doing it.'
(2) 'I absolutely should not have done the wrong thing.'
(3) 'Because I did what I absolutely should not have done, I am a sinner, a louse, a rotten person, who deserves to be punished.'

This trio, and this trio alone, is the essence of the feeling of guilt, sin and self-blame. The individual believes not only that he or she has done some wrong thing, committed some misdeed, or acted immorally towards some person or persons, but also that he or she is a worthless person for having done that wrong thing. The first statement may well be true. We need only establish what happened and who was harmed to secure agreement that some misdeed or immoral act was committed. Even if nobody was actually harmed, the individual could have broken a valued rule of personal conduct, and this, too, could be verified.

But what about the second statement? This is irrational because if you tell yourself that you *absolutely should not* have committed some misdeed when you actually did, you imply there is some law of the universe that states that you *must* not commit misdeeds. Now if such a law existed, you could not possibly act immorally, any more than you could break the law of gravity. It would make sense to say, 'I would prefer not to do the wrong thing', but when you use the words 'I *absolutely* should not', and really mean them, it makes no sense whatever. Can you, or anyone prove that any absolutes or cast-iron guarantees of morality actually exist in this world?

As for the third statement – which essentially is saying, 'I've turned into a rotten, damnable person because I did a wrong thing' – how could such a conclusion ever be verified scientifically? Moreover, the conclusion that you have become a rotten character who deserves to be punished is a *non sequitur* – it does not follow. For you could have said instead: 'I acted wrongly this time. Now how can I figure out ways of helping myself to act more ethically in future?' You could have said that; and saying it, and believing it, would help you to focus on the real problem of morality, namely, how to change your poor behaviour in future so that you act less immorally and relate in better ways to yourself and to other people. Whereas if you focus on self-condemnation and punishment, you will miss the real point: you will fail to *learn* from your various misdeeds and wrongdoing, and you will continue to perpetrate them indefinitely. You see, once you accept the concept of blame, and condemn and denigrate people for their wrongdoing, they will tend to consider themselves worthless and inadequate instead of merely mistaken or unethical. Then they will either go on the defensive and refuse to admit that what they did was wrong, or they will deny that they committed a wrong act in the first place. Consequently, they don't get around to the relatively simple act of acknowledging their errors and correcting them, because they become so preoccupied, due to their self-blame, with punishing themselves, or with denying that they did anything wrong at all. In other words, blame or guilt, instead of alleviating the amount of wrongdoing in the world, usually leads to more wrongdoing, hypocrisy and evasion of personal responsibility. To understand why condemning yourself for your misdeeds helps to *prevent* you from correcting your poor behaviour and making fewer errors in future, take the case of John, a young computer programmer.

A case of guilt

Using the A-B-C framework to illustrate our points is a good place to begin. By now, you may be becoming familiar with the model and the techniques employed and, hopefully, able to appreciate its advantages in clarifying the ways in which emotional disturbance arises.

John and Stephen share a flat in town. John, who is 25, does shift-work for a firm of computer software specialists, while Stephen, 23, works a straight nine-to-five day in a city office as a trainee accountant. One afternoon while in the flat alone, John noticed lying on the floor and partly hidden by the edge of the sofa, four £10 notes. Hanging above the sofa on a bracket on the wall, was one of Stephen's jackets. John realized that the money had probably dropped out of Stephen's jacket pocket. Being a bit short of cash as a result of paying a bit more than he intended for a new personal stereo, John put the £40 in his own pocket.

Later that evening, Stephen returned to the flat and told John he had lost £40 and that the money was probably lying somewhere in the flat. Together, they began to look for it, but after half an hour of fruitless search, Stephen concluded he must have dropped the money outside, a view with which John agreed. John felt relieved that Stephen did not suspect the money had been stolen, but his relief was short-lived. John felt no animosity towards Stephen; they had always got on well together. As the next few days went by, John became more and more morose and withdrawn. Stephen noticed the change in John and wondered what could have got into him. Soon, John became thoroughly depressed. As he told us later: 'I felt an absolute heel for the way I treated Stephen. It was bad enough to pinch his forty quid, but to kid him on I was looking for it when all the time I knew it was in my pocket, made me feel really rotten.'

In terms of our A-B-C model, at point A, John steals money belonging to Stephen and deceives him into thinking he has lost the money outside. At point C, John feels guilty and depressed. To feel that way, John would, according to our model, be holding both a rational and an irrational set of beliefs (at B) about what happened at A, the activating event.

Rationally, John believes: 'I acted wrongly in stealing money from my friend and deceiving him afterwards about it. How foolish of me to think that stealing Stephen's money would make up for my own financial shortsightedness! And now our friendship is not what it was. I would have acted more sensibly if I had owned up to Stephen and returned the money. That would have been the right thing to do, and even if he rejected me then, I could still accept myself.'

If John were to have stayed with that belief, his feelings at point C would be those of remorse and sorrow, and he would have felt able to return Stephen's money to him, and to resolve to be more self-disciplined about the management of his own finances in future.

Also at point B, John holds a different and much stronger set of beliefs about what happened at point A. It is this second set of evaluative conclusions about what happened which creates his strong feeling of guilt:

(1) 'I stole money from Stephen and deceived him to escape detection.'

(2) 'I absolutely should not have done what I knowingly did do.'
(3) 'I am a thoroughly rotten character and I ought to be punished.'

You will recognize from John's third statement that he is condemning or denigrating himself as a person and that this is the cause of his guilt. Self-denigration, you will recall from the previous chapter, is one of the quickest ways into depression. Behaviourally, John became withdrawn and avoided Stephen's company as much as possible. Soon, John developed a rash all over his body for which his doctor could find no medical explanation. Suspecting it was psychosomatic in origin, the doctor asked John if he was worried about something. John, of course, knew the answer but could not bring himself to admit it to his doctor. John dwelt incessantly upon his misdeed and upon what a rotten, loathsome person he had now become. One day, when driving to his office, he felt so miserable, that he failed to apply his usual concentration to his driving and collided with another vehicle and caused £500 worth of damage to his own and the other driver's vehicle. It was then that John came to seek help for his guilt.

Disputing guilt-inducing beliefs

John's counsellor quickly showed John how his guilt stemmed from his conviction that he *must not* act wrongly towards others, and that when he does so act (as he probably will from time to time because he is a fallible, error-prone human being), he is hardly so rotten he deserves to be condemned and roasted in hell. When you designate yourself a knave or despicable person for having committed an immoral act, although you can prove your act was immoral in the sense of unnecessarily harming someone, you can't prove *yourself* rotten. Your proposition 'I've turned into a real rotten character!' doesn't merely mean that *some* of your actions are immoral or harmful to others. It really means that, first, you have behaved badly; second, you will always behave badly, and cannot but act badly under any conceivable circumstances; and third, you deserve to be utterly condemned for allowing yourself to behave that way. Now, if you think about it, the first statement, that you have behaved badly, may be true. It could be substantiated by looking at the facts. But the second statement, that you cannot but act badly, is unprovable; for nobody can predict the future. That leaves the idea that you deserve utter condemnation. All one can say here is that this statement is an arbitrary definition, that it, too, is unprovable, and that it is harm-creating because it diverts you from facing the real problem of how to behave less immorally in future.

At first, John had a hard time in accepting these arguments. Like most people, he had been brought up to believe that when he did wrong, that made him a sinner, that he and his acts, traits and characteristics were one and the same thing. 'Imagine I gave you a basket of fruit', said John's counsellor. 'In this basket are various fruits. Some, like these peaches, are in good condition, ripe, juicy and good for eating. Others, like these apples, are a bit blemished and not so good for eating, while one or two other fruits are spotty with rotten areas you can clearly see. Now, the question is this: is your basket a good basket, because it has some good fruit in it, or is it a bad basket because it contains some not so good fruit?' Being an intelligent fellow, John saw the point, and replied: 'Well, it's neither. Having some ripe fruit in it doesn't make it a good basket, any more than those blemished apples in it make it a bad basket. It's just a basket.' The counsellor then went on to explain to John in more detail why it is invalid to label himself, or anyone else for that matter, as a villain or wicked person for behaving wickedly. Let's consider these reasons now at greater length.

You and your acts are not the same thing

First, as we have already pointed out, if you were a bad, wicked person for behaving badly, you would always and could only act badly. The implication here is that you are intrinsically bad or wicked and that you have no redeeming features whatsoever. It means that no matter how many years you lived, you could only continue to perform bad or wicked deeds. How could this ever be proved? If we humans were pre-programmed robots, so that we could act only in certain ways, the statement could logically at least make some sense – although even robots can sometimes behave differently from their design specifications! On the other hand, we do not appear to have unlimited free will, but we do have some degree of freedom of choice in deciding how to run our lives. Given that, we contend that no matter how many times you were to act badly, the fact that you are a live human being in this world and have the power of choice, means that you could *choose* to change your wicked behaviour, and cease to carry out wicked acts. Even Hitler and Stalin, who between them were responsible, directly and indirectly, for genocide on a huge scale, and who perpetrated some of the most appalling acts of cruelty against human beings the world had ever known, were not 100 per cent evil. They appear to have possessed *some* good points – not many, but one or two!

Second, if you label a person who acts wickedly as a totally worthless creature you are implying that this person is *fully* responsible for his or her actions and therefore deserves severe punishment and total condemnation for acting badly. But a person who *consistently* acts badly may well be found to have pronouced hereditary and/or environmentally acquired tendencies to behave that way, through a very poor upbringing, for instance, allied to a strong genetic disposition. How then, can that person be held *totally* responsible, far less damnable, for character traits which were inborn or acquired from childhood onwards?

Third, when an individual is labelled 'no good', either by himself, or by others for his poor behaviour or misdeeds, the error being made here is the assumption that the individual is the same thing as his behaviour. On the basis of this (erroneous) assumption, people tend to label themselves as 'good' when they perform well at various tasks (such as winning approval from others), and to rate themselves as 'bad' whenever they do poorly. We have already (in the previous chapter), given you several reasons why you cannot legitimately rate yourself in terms of your behaviour; in view of their importance in helping you to acquire a philosophy of self-acceptance as distinct from an attitude of self-rating, we make no apology for repeating the substance of these arguments here.

How to stop labelling yourself

We are complex human beings with an enormous number of traits, characteristics and mannerisms. Moreover, these traits and abilities change as you go through life; they are not static entities. You can give these various traits a rating depending upon how well they help you achieve your personal goals. For example, you might say, 'I have lots of patience with children and I get on well with them.' You could evaluate that trait as good if you were planning to become a child-minder or a primary school teacher. Or, you might be very studious and able to devote long hours each night to studying books. That trait, too, could be rated good if you were planning on becoming a lawyer or accountant. However, if your goal were to become a professional boxer, your studious inclinations might not be rated highly at all. Your deeds, acts and personality characteristics are only aspects of you; they are not your totality. What we call the 'self' is really an ongoing ever-changing *process* that has a past, present and future and that, therefore, cannot legitimately be rated or measured in any once-and-for-all manner. Neither you, nor anyone else, can ever give you a global report card. Your identity, your essence, is irreducible and cannot be labelled or graded in a way that would make any sense. When you consider that the average person fulfils in his or her lifetime many roles in society, with varying degrees of competence and success, it is clear that no conceivable system of measurement could come to grips with a demand to rate that person as 'good' or 'bad'. What is the solution? Obviously, don't rate yourself at all. Assess your abilities and deeds as good or bad, if you will, but remember, a good deed no more makes you a good person than a bad deed makes you a bad person. Since you have no overall worth, neither have you any overall worthlessness. Human worth and worthlessness are definitions or concepts which we have made up ourselves and which are vague and quite unrelated to reality. It follows that whenever you censure your*self*, blame your*self* or loathe your*self* for acting badly, either in your own eyes or in those of someone else, you are really demeaning your*self*, your *essence* or soul, for your unfortunate deeds.

Accept yourself – unconditionally

Full self-acceptance, then, or what the famous American psychologist, Carl Rogers, called 'unconditional positive regard', is probably the one quality you need more than almost anything else for a happy existence. For not only will you find it difficult to denigrate yourself when you behave less well than you might, or when other people withhold their approval of your behaviour, but you will be more highly motivated to eliminate your needless anxiety about your future actions, and to work constructively to improve both your behaviour and your relations with other people. If you choose only to accept yourself when you act well and competently, or when you win other people's approval, you set yourself up for potential feelings of non-self-acceptance when you don't do so well (as will sometimes happen), and when you fail to gain the approval of others (which can also frequently happen). Unconditional self-acceptance will give you virtually a head start in eliminating the various roadblocks to the happier, more pleasurable existence you could have; and the beauty of it is it's yours for the asking.

Thus far, we have tried to show you that feelings of guilt arise from irrational, condemnatory self-evaluations following the commission of some misdeed, and that if you truly accept yourself as a fallible, error-prone human being who will never be perfect, you will not inevitably *feel* guilty (that is, self-deprecating) whenever you perform some act which violates your moral standards. In other words, there is a rational alternative to guilt, which we will now describe.

The rational alternative to guilt

It is an observed fact that society changes only slowly in response to changes in our knowledge and understanding of the world. It takes time for modern ideas on the treatment of delinquent children and adults to percolate through to those institutions responsible for the administration of justice, for example. More realistic ideas on marriage, divorce and contraception have gained acceptance only after decades of persistent challenging of antiquated notions handed down from the past. Not surprisingly, our society is still wedded to ancient views on crime and punishment which originated long before the advent of modern psychological knowledge began to give us some understanding of what makes human beings 'tick'. We still tend to hold people fully responsible for their crimes and misdeeds and demand that they be blamed and punished until they have atoned for their wrongdoing. And we are brought up and taught to blame ourselves and to expect punishment when we do wrong things. It is very doubtful if this punitive philosophy actually promotes more moral behaviour. We shall deal with this important matter presently. For the moment, let us show you what we mean by a rational alternative to guilt.

First of all, acknowledge your wrongdoing or immorality. Don't hide behind excuses or try to explain it away. If you steal from someone, acknowledge your responsibility for your act. Returning to the example we gave you earlier, when John eventually changed his irrational beliefs, he was able to say to himself: 'Yes, I stole money from Stephen. I committed that offence and I realize I behaved wrongly.' That is a sane and factual observation. 'Now,' continued John's counsellor, 'what would you follow with? How would you continue? Would you tell yourself over and over again, "Oh, what a villain I am for doing that to Stephen! However will I live this down?" ' 'No', replied John. 'Well, what would you say, instead?' asked the counsellor. 'I committed a wrong against Stephen. How can I make amends to him, and how can I prevent myself from doing a wrong deed again; that is my answer', replied John. 'That's better', said the counsellor. 'Provided you concentrate on how to change your poor behaviour in the future instead of bemoaning your past misdeeds, you will improve your chances of working out how to behave less immorally in the future. Go to Stephen and tell him what you did. Return his money to him and apologize for your behaviour. Offer to do something for him for inconveniencing him. You will have a better chance of repairing your broken relationship with him than if you desperately beg his forgiveness or try to punish yourself in some way.' The point here is that you cannot undo what has undoubtedly been done. If you have harmed someone, sensibly resolve to help the person in the present and in the future. Realize that you should behave morally towards others because it is in your own best interests to do so. If you needlessly harm others or act selfishly and inconsiderately towards them, you will frequently encourage them to pay you back in kind. What good will that do you? You behave in accordance with the moral rules and precepts of your community, not because you see yourself as a worm or sinner when you don't, but because, in the final analysis, you will harm yourself and those you love if you violate the rights of others, or behave nastily and unfairly towards them. 'Do unto others as you would be done by' is still a golden rule to live by.

Even if you are now convinced that guilt feelings are essentially irrational, you may possibly be of the opinion that severely blaming and censuring wrongdoers for their misdeeds will at least help to stop them from committing quite so many crimes in future. 'If we never blamed anybody for their immoral or criminal deeds, wouldn't that just encourage people to go on behaving badly, and to think it didn't matter when they did wrong?' you may ask. Well, our contention is that blaming wrongdoers for their wrong acts is not merely unhelpful in reducing the amount of immoral or criminal behaviour in society, but in some ways makes the commission of wrongful deeds even more likely. So, to see how this comes about, let us examine in some detail the social consequences of blaming people for their mistaken behaviour.

Why guilt won't make you a happy, healthy, law-abiding citizen

We have tried, in the above paragraphs, to show you that feelings of guilt or self-blame are derived from irrational and unsustainable ideas. On logical and empirical grounds, that is to say, they are unrealistic and untenable. If that was all, guilt would scarcely exist as a major problem; the sheer discomfort of carrying guilty feelings around with nothing to show for it would tend to be seen as a fairly pointless sort of activity. Unfortunately, the deliberate inculcation by the media of feelings of guilt, sin and self-blame and even blame of others in those regarded as responsible for various kinds of wrongdoing, is something of a growth industry these days. Whenever some disaster occurs which appears to be due to human error, almost the first question to be raised is 'Who is to blame for it?' Not 'Who is responsible for it?' but 'Whom can we blame for this?' It is almost as if *we* will feel better about the consequences of a disaster if we can fasten some blame on *someone else*. Such a punitive philosophy helps to make people feel enormously guilty (rather than sincerely sorry) about many of the things they do which are considered wrong; not only that, feelings of guilt frequently lead to anxiety, depression and hostility as well as pronounced feelings of inadequacy and self-hatred.

Does guilt ever help?

In view of the near universality of the use of guilt as a means of getting us to act more normally, can anything be said for it? In our view, very little! While it would be inaccurate to claim that giving human beings a sense of sin, guilt or self-blame for their misdeeds *never* helps them to correct their mistaken or criminal behaviour, the results can be exceedingly unhelpful. It may work with many children because they tend to be highly suggestible. It may even work with some adults, for the same reason. But only for a time! Even when blame is effective, and people commit fewer misdeeds because of harsh punishment and social sanctions levelled against them during their formative years, their conformity with the rules of social living tends to be accompanied with feelings of fear and resentment. Such feelings are hardly conducive to enabling people freely and voluntarily to adopt the highest standards of personal or social behaviour. In fact, when people are savagely denounced for their misdeeds they may be made to toe the line for fear of further punishment being meted out to them, but the toll in terms of the emotional turmoil suffered – the intense degrees of guilt and anxiety that are built up – is so great as to make one doubt the value of what little amount of moral behaviour is thereby achieved.

Still another consequence of self-blame can be seen in the case of those individuals who have an acute sense of sin. Whenever they feel impelled at times to commit wrong deeds (which they often do), their sense of sin and the merciless self-blame that accompanies it result in a deep sense of worthlessness. The full realization of deep worthlessness is so severe an insult to the 'ego' that the wrongdoer reacts by either denying to himself (repressing) all thoughts about his wrongdoing or insisting that he did not do any wrong.

Still others in a self-condemnatory frame of mind attempt to anaesthetize themselves from the pain of guilt by resorting to over-indulgence in alcohol or the consumption of drugs. The effects of such attempts to escape from guilt only deepen the feelings of worthlessness which were there in the first place and a vicious circle of self-loathing and escapism is set in motion which may result in the hospitalization of the individual, or even in suicide. As you saw earlier in the case of John, telling yourself what a villain you are for behaving badly and strongly believing you deserve to be punished, can become a self-fulfilling prophecy; the rash of spots on his body and subsequent mishap with his car stemmed directly from his state of mind. There is a saying in the Talmud: 'God may forgive you for your sins, your nervous system won't.' You would do well to remember it! In any case, punishing yourself implies that the punishment will do some good – will help to right the wrong, or make it less likely that you will do wrong again. It is obvious that no matter how much you punish yourself, the person you harmed will reap no benefit from it. And if you look at the history of human punishment and check it against what happens in the world today, you will find it difficult to maintain that condemning and punishing people for their sins effectively prevents them from doing wicked things again. No group has been more condemned and hated than the IRA. Yet, in spite of all the condemnation and the punishment meted out to various members of that group, they still continue with unabated ferocity to blow up and gun down anyone they think stands in the way of achieving their aims.

Even when an individual with self-punishing tendencies tries to make amends for his or her misdeeds, the results often fall far short of the person's expectations. As has aptly been noted in a recent publication:

> Typically in guilt, since the person is in a self-condemnatory frame of mind, she is likely to choose options from her response repertoire which tend to make it more likely that she will 'sin' in future. For example, a common pattern in eating disorders involves the person resolving to diet, establishing a strict dieting regime, breaking this regime, condemning herself, and eating to take away the pain of guilt. If the person experiencing guilt considers that she has wronged another, she is likely to make unrealistic promises to the other to the effect that 'I will never do that again', without attempting to understand the factors which led her to act that way. She thus finds it difficult to learn from her errors, and thus tends not to be able to keep such promises. Thus, people who experience guilt are often so preoccupied with 'purging' their badness, or with self-punishment, that they tend not to look for explanations for their behaviour other than those that involve internal attributions of badness.*

We might add, too, that in some instances, when people label themselves as rotten villains for doing rotten or wicked acts, they believe they are compelled to act badly in future, because that is what being a villain really means, and thus they become compulsive wrongdoers.

These, then, are some reasons why, almost inevitably, giving people a sense of guilt or self-worthlessness when they perform criminal or immoral acts will not make for less wrongdoing or improve the moral tone or mental health of society. What, then, can we do to help people change their poor behaviour instead of punishing them – or encouraging them to punish themselves?

*W. Dryden, *Counselling Individuals: The Rational-Emotive Approach* (Taylor & Francis, 1987)

You can help create a saner society

Let us make one thing very clear: we are emphatically *not* suggesting that people should be encouraged to take a 'so what?' or 'couldn't care less' attitude to their own misdeeds and wrongdoing. Along with sane-thinking persons throughout the world, we accept that, as members of a social group, as citizens of a social community which itself is part of a world community, we must have *some* standards of right and wrong if we wish to live in a civilized manner and pursue our personal aims in life. We believe that wrongdoers should be *penalized* – not punished – for their misdeeds, and that penal institutions could best serve the interests of society, and of wrongdoers, if such institutions were places where psycho-educational programmes of rehabilitation were attempted, rather than merely places where one 'does time'. We attach importance to teaching basic moral principles to children and young people and to showing them why it is in their own best interest to act fairly and considerately towards others, while still primarily seeking to achieve their own goals in life. We mentioned the importance of standards. Our own view is that these standards are based on long-range hedonism – that is, the philosophy that one may strive primarily for the achievement of one's own goals and satisfactions in life, while at the same time bearing in mind that one will achieve one's best results in most cases by giving up immediate gratifications for future gains and by being courteous and considerate to others. If we ride roughshod over other people's desires to achieve their goals and satisfactions, we will usually sabotage our own ends. Almost any rationally planned and democratically acceptable set of moral rules would be OK.

Life without guilt

The fundamental problem of human morality is not the problem of appeasing some hypothetical deity because we may have committed some act which incurs the wrath of the deity; nor is it the problem of punishing ourselves for our mistakes, acts or misdeeds. Rather, the basic problem is the very simple one of teaching a person not to commit an anti-social act in the first place, and, if he does commit it, teaching him to acknowledge he has done it and to learn how not to commit it again in the second place. This problem could be solved if potential or actual wrongdoers were taught to believe 'If I carry out this act it will be wrong' and to ask themselves 'How do I act so as to avoid doing this wrong?' Or to tell themselves 'This deed I have done is wrong and harmful to others' and to ask 'Now how do I act so that I do *not* do this wrong act again?'

In other words, you acknowledge your wrongdoing or immorality.

Thus, if you needlessly harm another person (for example, by stealing from or physically hurting him or her), acknowledge your responsibility for the act. Say to yourself: 'Yes, I committed that offence. It was wrong of me.' Then, instead of saying, 'I must label myself a villain or louse who deserves punishment for this deed', you say: 'Alright, I did the wrong thing this time. Now, how can I make amends to this person for my misdeed, but more especially how can I figure out how *not* to do such a mistaken thing again?' In short, without any self-condemnation, resolve sensibly, now and in the future, to help the person you have harmed and to refrain from harming him or her again. We contend that when these ideas really become part of you, you will find it hard to commit or keep committing immoral acts.

Why people do wrong

When people perform acts which they or others consider wrong or immoral, they do so, in the final analysis, because they are too stupid, too ignorant, or too emotionally disturbed to refrain from doing so. While such people undoubtedly cause harm to, or are responsible for harming others, it is illogical to denigrate them as human beings for their stupidity, ignorance or disturbance. We contend that the only basic solution to the problem of emotional disturbance is the correction or cessation of the disturbed person's anti-social actions. This can be effected only if we give the disturbed person insight into the 'hows' and 'whys' of his mistaken and self-defeating behaviour and provide him with a highly effective active programme of working at the eradication of his behaviour. In the case of psychopaths and politically motivated wrongdoers, if we had our way (which seems very unlikely!) we would institutionalize these people for a sufficiently long period of re-education, to try to recover some elements of their humanity in the hope that one day they would be able to lead more sensible, less hate-filled lives. The psycho-educational techniques are available for this enterprise; the political will to use them is not. Too many institutions and organizations would lose their credibility, and therefore their power over people, if the concept of sin and blame were abandoned by a significant number of human beings.

In passing, we would mention that we are aware that some of our politically-minded friends would argue that the best way, perhaps the only way, to change society, is to start at the top and work down to bring about the changes we want. By all means, try it! One disadvantage of this approach is that it requires a political party with enough power and internal cohesion to carry out the desired changes. But as we know, political parties can split up and change their policies and priorities.

They depend upon sufficient consensus (at least in democratic societies) to carry out their programmes. Since we cannot control how others think or decide what is important for them, it may be that our best bet is to start with ourselves. After all, we *can* change how *we* think and feel! And if a sufficient number of us were to abandon the concept of guilt and adopt the rational alternative to guilt set out in this book, who knows what changes for the best might not come about as a result? Be that as it may, we firmly maintain that if we can teach people the world over that, even though they can be quite accountable or responsible for their misdeeds, no one is ever to *blame* for anything he does, then human morality will be significantly improved and, for the first time in the history of our world, civilized people will have a real chance to achieve and maintain mental health. The sooner we learn to eliminate guilt using the techniques of identifying and disputing the irrationality of blaming oneself and others, and augmenting these with other ways of changing our irrational beliefs as set out in this book, the better our world will be.

SUMMARY POINTS FOR CHAPTER 4

(1) When you feel guilty over having committed some misdeed, or over having failed to meet some ethical standard, there are two components to how you see your situation. First, you are aware of having transgressed some code of moral behaviour. Then you condemn yourself for having done so.

(2) Your acknowledgement of wrongdoing (assuming that you actually did, or are continuing to do, the wrong thing) is rational in that you take responsibility for your own behaviour, and this may help you to change your immoral behaviour in future.

(3) Unfortunately, when you go on to condemn yourself as a sinner or a rotten person for having done the wrong thing, the chances are you will continue to act wrongly. Once you accept that you are blameworthy and damnable for having acted badly, you will see yourself as worthless and inadequate, instead of merely mistaken or unethical. Then you will either defensively refuse to admit that what you did was wrong, or even deny that you committed a misdeed in the first place.

(4) Unhelpful as the feeling of guilt is in helping you recognize your wrongdoing and behave more morally in future, guilt also stems from two deeply irrational beliefs. These are:

(a) 'I absolutely should not have done the wrong thing.'
(b) 'Because I did what I absolutely should not have done, I am a sinner, a louse, a rotten person who deserves to be punished.'

(5) Using the A-B-C model, we showed you in detail how to dispute these irrational beliefs and replace them with more rational ones. We paid special attention to the idea that the 'self' cannot be rated or measured in any way, and that you are not the same thing as your deeds or traits; these may be given a rating, but your *self* cannot.

(6) Having argued for the need for some generally accepted standards of right and wrong behaviour in civilized society if we wish to live in peace and pursue our aims in life, we showed that the concept of guilt is not only self-defeating but socially unhelpful as well.

(7) Finally, we put forward a rational alternative to guilt and urged you to abandon the concept of guilt and sin to give yourselves a real chance to raise the level of mental health in society and to live more sanely and enjoyably.

5

Anger and Hostility

Some thirty or so years ago, a song with the title 'Love and Marriage' became very popular. Some of you may remember it: the tune was catchy and the words went something like this: 'Love and marriage, love and marriage, go together like a horse and carriage', and it ended with the refrain 'You can't have one without the other'. Even for the 1950s that last line was something of a rash promise. Today, it would probably make the *Guinness Book of Records* under the heading 'How wrong can you be?' That famous duo, love and marriage, still continues to weave its spell today, although we have noticed that the first member of the pair quite often prefers to consort with other partners instead of, and sometimes in addition to, its more usual companion, marriage! If the composer of 'Love and Marriage' had been around today, we might have persuaded him that if he was looking for a permanent couple to write a song about, he could do no better than to select the title of this chapter. If we may paraphrase that last line of the song 'Love and Marriage' to tie in with anger and hostility, it would read 'If you have the one, you can hardly avoid the other!' Anger and hostility are a couple, who, unlike love and marriage, ought to be separated and their relationship dissolved for the simple reason that the cost of maintaining them is enormous. We will show you why in a moment. Before we do so, however, it will be instructive to take a look at one or two popular folk remedies which have been put forward as a way of dealing with this unhappy couple. You will then be in a position to compare the effectiveness of these remedies with our Rational-Emotive Therapy (RET) approach to the problem of anger and hostility. But first, what do we mean by 'anger'?

Is anger the same as annoyance?

Some of you may ask: 'Isn't anger just the same thing as great annoyance? If someone treats me unfairly, or carelessly damages some valuable possession of mine, am I not entitled to feel very annoyed or angry with that person?' Our answer is that you would justifiably feel annoyed or intensely displeased, but angry – no! Anger is *not* the same as intense displeasure or great annoyance. Consider this: with a bit of effort, you can conceal your annoyance when you think it may be wiser not to display it. It is an entirely different matter to pretend you don't feel angry when you really are angry, because the physiological changes which accompany anger are visible and give you away. Your blood pressure builds up, you turn red in the face, you tremble as the adrenalin pours into your bloodstream to prepare your whole body for an emergency. It is a very uncomfortable feeling and it is dangerous. Apart from the harm it may do to you, anger may well lead to violence against others. The violent society is the end result when enough people practise violence as a way of life when confronted with the inevitable frustrations we all encounter in our daily living. If you wanted to make this world a less violent and happier place to live in, wouldn't you think it worth learning how to diminish hate and anger by becoming a sane, unangry person yourself? You have nothing to lose by trying, and the reduced strain on your internal physiological system from learning to live without anger may even add a few years to your life. Annoyance, irritation and displeasure you can expect. It is healthy to feel annoyed or irritated when some person or some circumstance stands in the way of your attaining some objective. For then, rationally, you can say: 'I do not like this situation, and I intend to change it if I can in order to achieve my aim.' Your disliking something motivates you to change it. If you had no feelings at all when your wishes remained unfulfilled, it is doubtful if you could survive for long in this 'desireless' state! The feeling of discomfort you get when your wishes are frustrated can encourage you to continue to strive assertively to protect your own interests instead of just giving up, while also acknowledging the right of others to strive for what they consider is in their best interests. So annoyance is a normal part of living. But that fist-clenching, gut-wrenching, trembling feeling that we call anger is bad for you and for society. We will now show you how anger is created and how you can eliminate or reduce it to the point where it need never bother you again.

Most people today, when faced with the frustrations and hassles of everyday life, assume that you can hardly avoid feeling angry when blocked from achieving what you see are your legitimate aims and goals in life. We have no choice, it seems, but to feel angry when people treat us unfairly, cause us considerable inconvenience through their negligence and stupidity, or interfere in some way with our plans. That may be most people's view, including some psychologists'; it certainly isn't ours. Few psychologists understand the latest psychological findings on the nature of anger. The general public, therefore, can hardly be expected to know any better. The ideas we shall present to you are very unusual, and yet very effective and relatively quick when they are understood and practised, and we will shortly explain them to you as simply and as clearly as we can. But before we begin, let's take a brief look at some of the popular suggestions and exhortations proffered to us in numerous books, magazine articles and sermons.

Unhelpful ways of dealing with anger

Squelch your anger

Here you feel your anger but don't express it. You bottle it up, put the lid on it. In this way you avoid an angry confrontation – but at what cost! It's rather like a pressure cooker. Keeping your feelings pent up inside isn't going to help you dissipate your anger. The more often you suppress your anger, the more likely it is that some day you are going to lose control and let your anger explode. If, on the other hand, you do manage to keep the lid down on your anger, you won't necessarily feel better. You can't hide your anger away. It stays right there inside you, simmering away, and one day you're going to wonder what's giving you stomach ulcers, high blood pressure, migraines and other psychosomatic symptoms. On top of that, you may start to blame yourself for not standing up for yourself when others treat you unfairly. And if you've read the previous chapter on guilt, you'll know how little good self-blame will do you! 'OK', you might say. 'How about expressing our anger openly when we are unjustly treated? Letting people know about our feelings, letting all that pent up feeling come right out – boy, I can just picture the look on certain people's faces if I came out with it and told them what I *really* think about them! You won't get migraines and all that other stuff now, will you?' Perhaps not, we would answer. But why not take a good look at what you *will* get when you give free vent to your feelings?

Freely express your anger: letting it all hang out

Suppose you feel really angry with someone and you let that person know how you feel. Most people would feel good about expressing their self-righteous indignation over some wrong or injustice they had suffered. But what effect do you think it will have on those on the receiving end of your bitter, acccusing words? Nine times out of ten, they will resent your expression of anger and interpret it as an aggressive and hostile act on your part. They will then defensively withdraw from you or react to your barrage with their own hostility. Either way, you will get no satisfaction from the other person; for even if he or she was inclined to consider apologizing for his or her behaviour towards you, once you angrily confront that person your anger and perceived hostility will drive away any thought the other person may have had of reaching some kind of understanding with you. Thus you defeat yourself in the end because you wind up with the same situation as before you angrily blew your top. Nothing will have been resolved by your angry outburst; indeed, the situation may have been made worse and a satisfactory solution to your disagreement made even more unlikely.

A variation to expressing your anger verbally and directly to someone is to use the technique supposedly favoured by Japanese executives when the stresses they experience through working with difficult people tend to surface in angry words. The enraged executive is placed in a room with pillows and pummels and punches the pillows while simultaneously imagining he is punching some hated boss or customer. He continues with the punching and the name-calling under these 'safe' conditions until the pent-up feelings of anger presumably are dissipated.

You might think this is a good idea because it is safe and harmless; only the pillows get punched, and pillows can't punch back! True enough, but the consequences are not so harmless. So long as the angry individual feels good as he pounds away at the pillow, he will tend to reinforce his propensity to anger because he derives such pleasure from expressing it later in the pillow room. Thus the angry individual has no incentive to work at undoing his anger-creating philosophy since he knows that he will derive some pleasure from pounding the pillows which represent for him the various people he is angry with. All he needs to do when he feels angry is to hold his anger in check until he can make it to the pillow room. In other words, providing a safe outlet for your anger will practically guarantee that you will never get around to looking at ways of living without anger.

Creative aggression: let's both express
our anger to each other

The idea behind creative aggression or 'constructive anger', as it is called, is that you agree beforehand with the person you feel angry with, to have a session during which each person gives the other 'permission' to vent his or her true feelings about the matter under contention. Presumably this clears the air between the antagonists and appears to have some merit in that each person is prepared to listen to the other's angry tirade without feeling surprised or put at a disadvantage by the verbal attacks, as they might in a confrontation that has not been prearranged.

It is claimed that this method works best with people who know each other well, such as married couples, family members and other types of close associates. Creative aggression might work in some cases where the couple concerned can take it; in other cases it might not work at all. You can never be sure how someone, even someone you know well, will react to a verbal onslaught, especially if the recipient feels very defensive and vulnerable to certain criticisms. In any case, neither this, nor the preceding techniques for dealing with the expression of angry feelings, really help people understand how their anger is created in the first place. These methods all tacitly assume what most people throughout the world mistakenly believe: that their angry feelings are created by others or by frustrating circumstances. We will discuss just one other method of responding to anger before we get down to showing you how your angry feelings are really created and how you can eradicate them and lead a calmer existence, regardless of your personal circumstances.

The placid approach

'A soft answer turneth away wrath', says the Bible. If you find yourself at the receiving end of some person's angry words, keeping your mouth shut, or permitting yourself only the occasional innocuous remark may well prevent an outburst of anger. At first, the other person may become even more enraged at your failure to respond as he or she expects. But after a relatively short time, the other person will give up when he realizes you are not going to play his game. So this method has some merit in that it helps to de-escalate a potentially angry build-up. Its disadvantage is that the other person may interpret your lack of response to his angry criticisms as a sign that you don't really care enough for your own interest, or that you are unwilling to stand up for it. The consequence is that others, noticing your passive behaviour, may think they can ignore your wants and take advantage of your good nature.

All in all, we think some of these techniques will work for some people, some of the time, but that none of them will help anyone to live unangrily for very long. The reason is that none of these methods really uncover the root causes of anger. It stands to reason that if people are unaware of the fundamental cause of a problem, they are unlikely to find the solution to it. The various ways of responding to anger described above are essentially palliative solutions; that is, they may, at best, achieve some short-term improvement, but they can never produce any real long-lasting gains and consequently are largely ineffective in offering people a way of eliminating their anger without losing their will to strive for what they really want out of life. We will now show you an entirely new approach to this age-old problem of anger, an approach which has been scientifically tried and tested and which you can master and use to enhance your own happiness and that of your loved ones.

You make yourself angry

The RET approach to anger is the same approach as we have used in indentifying anxiety, guilt and depression, which we have already outlined in previous chapters. RET consistently states that if you want to change some damaging or fruitless emotion or behaviour, and to do so in the quickest and most efficient manner possible, you are advised to change your belief system. Other people or difficult circumstances in your life don't *make* you angry; *you* do! Other people and difficult circumstances may contribute to your upset feelings, but it is your own self-defeating beliefs about other people's actions, or about the frustrating conditions of your life which really do the damage. The Greek philosopher, Epictetus, put it this way nearly 2000 years ago: 'Since you think your way into emotional turmoil, it follows that you can think your way out of it.' Let's turn our attention now to showing you how to identify your anger-creating philosophies and how to use the RET method to rip them up.

The A-B-C of anger

We begin by recognizing that most people have goals in life. Generally, people the world over do what they think they have to do in order to survive, and to survive as happily, or at least as pain-free, as they can. Different cultures also emphasize their own ideas as to what their members ought to do and ought not to do. In our own society, for example, we attach importance to education, getting a good job with interesting work, raising a family and many other activities which we share with others to a large extent. We all have our own desires and wishes but will probably realize only a fraction of them in our lifetime. We cannot have all we want because life itself frustrates many of our goals. There are limits to our time, our efforts and our resources. Not getting all, or even most, of what we want from life is an unavoidable regret. If we are wise, we accept these inevitable frustrations of life, while actively disliking them, even as we strive to gain through our hard work as much as we can of our dreams. So we are frustrated in achieving many of our goals in life. But does the frustration make us angry? A few years ago some psychologists thought so. They called it the frustration –aggression hypothesis. These psychologists confirmed the teaching of society, of parents, and of teachers, that being frustrated must lead to aggression – frustration makes you angry. It causes you to become angry. Let's see if this idea really holds water.

At point A we have some activating event. Let us suppose you have arranged with a maintenance engineer to visit your home at a mutually agreed date and time to overhall your central heating system. You have explained to the engineer that you will take time off work that day at your own expense to remain at home so as to be there when he arrives to carry out the work. The engineer estimates the work will require two or three hours of his time and he gives you a firm assurance that he will be at your home on that date and at a mutually agreed time. When the day arrives he fails to turn up. You receive no phone call or other communication to explain his non-appearance. In addition, you have lost a day's work and a day's pay. At point C, the emotional consequence, you feel decidedly angry. You mentally rehearse in your mind how you are going to 'tear him off a strip' when you get hold of him. Your anger has ruined your appetite and your only thought is how you are going to get even with the man for having 'caused' you to waste your whole day.

According to RET, you have both appropriate and inappropriate feelings about the things that happen to you. Appropriate feelings stem from appraisals of your situation which help you to attain your objectives or deal with obstacles in such a way as to minimize feeling needless emotional pain when you are prevented from getting what you want. By contrast, inappropriate feelings inhibit you from attaining your objectives and sabotage your attempts to cope with the situation constructively. They tend, in fact, to make it worse. As we have maintained throughout this book, your feelings, appropriate and inappropriate, are created by your beliefs and evaluations about the happenings in your life. Thus, at point B, you have two sets of beliefs: a set of rational beliefs leading to appropriate feelings and behaviours; and a set of irrational beliefs leading to inappropriate, self-defeating feelings and behaviours. Now, what do these beliefs consist of?

First, take your rational beliefs about the engineer not turning up when he said he would. You correctly observe that you have been inconvenienced by his failure to appear at the agreed time. You have lost money and no doubt another day's pay will be lost when you succeed in making a second appointment with the engineer to overhaul your domestic heating system. You say to yourself: 'By not turning up and not letting me know why, he has placed me in an awkward situation. I'll have to arrange another date for him to come over and that means a further loss of income to me. How annoying! I wish he had turned up on time.' If you stayed with that belief about the situation you would feel merely displeased, irritated and annoyed, but not angry.

Why is this belief rational? First, it is factual. You can prove that you have been inconvenienced and put to some unforeseen expense. Almost anyone looking at your situation would agree that you had a right to feel disappointed and displeased. Second, your displeasure at being inconvenienced will encourage you to confront the engineer and calmly ask him for an explanation for his failure to keep his part of the agreement. By doing so, you might be able to negotiate a reduction in his fee to compensate you for the day's pay you have lost. Thus, your rational beliefs about your frustrating situation generate appropriate feelings of annoyance, which in turn motivate you to take some constructive action to safeguard your own interests in a manner more likely to be acceptable to the other person than if you angrily condemned him for his failure to keep to the agreement.

Now let's look at your irrational beliefs. You actually *are* feeling angry, and you have spent the rest of the day fuming over the engineer's 'inconsiderateness' and sheer gall in treating you this way, especially after he had promised you he would be there when you agreed it with him. What sort of things are going through your mind and creating your decidedly angry mood? In all probability, you would be saying something like:

(1) 'How *awful* of him not to turn up when he said he would and to treat me so unfairly!'
(2) 'I *can't stand* it when people treat me in such an irresponsible and unjust manner!'
(3) 'He *should not* and *must not* behave like that towards me, especially after promising me that he would turn up on time.'
(4) 'He *deserves to be condemned and punished* for acting so inconsiderately towards me!'

We hope you can see the reason why all four of these statements are irrational. You are essentially saying: 'Because the engineer acted unfairly and inconsiderately towards me, which he should not have done, he is a bad person.' The major error here is to equate the person with his behaviour. Granted, for the sake of argument, that he behaved badly towards you, how does that alone make him a bad person? He might not have acted badly towards you. For all you know, he might have left to keep his appointment with you and subsequently been involved in a traffic accident which made it impossible for him to contact you. You merely inferred that the engineer's failure to arrive was due to inconsiderate behaviour on his part. But even if it was a deliberate act of neglect to keep his appointment, how does that make him a bad person? As we showed you in Chapter 3, when you equate a person with his or her actions, you are implying that all bad acts can only be performed by bad people, that only a bad person can perform bad deeds. Conversely, by the same token, all good acts can only be performed by good people and only a good person can perform good deeds. Is this true in fact?

If you believe this to be true, you will find it easy to view a person as bad if that person does something which runs counter to your personal beliefs on what is right and what is wrong. If, further, you believe that he or she absolutely *should not* transgress against your own personal rules of conduct, then when they do, on occasion, do just that, you will condemn them and try to punish them for their action. If this, in turn, leads to physical violence against the transgressor of your rules, you may land yourself in serious trouble. If you content yourself by carrying out an angry confrontation with the person you are blaming, you are unlikely to achieve the goal you first set out to achieve; at the end of the day, your heating system will still be in a state of disrepair. Your anger will have got you nowhere and you will be the loser. Does anger, then, never do you any good? Sometimes it can, but not very often! If your life is threatened and you are cornered and there is no way out for you except to fight, then anger can give you that extra strength to help you fight or escape. But unless you are very unfortunate, you will seldom encounter such life and death situations. Weigh up the costs of anger, to yourself as well as to your loved ones and you will realize why anger can seldom by justified. Dr Paul Hauck, an esteemed colleague of ours, claims that anger is the greatest single cause of divorce.* Not money, or sex, or in-laws, or other women, but anger. Dr Hauck's book is entirely about anger and how to eradicate it from your life. It is packed with sage advice and we highly recommend it to anyone who is troubled with anger.

Now look again at what your underlying philosophy is when you condemn someone for breaking some personal rule of yours. This can be seen quite clearly from this irrational idea: 'He *should not* and *must not* behave like that towards me, especially after promising me.' If you believe that idea you are demanding that other people obey your rules and that they have no right to be wrong. Since nobody is perfect, and since we all make innumerable mistakes throughout the course of our lives because we are fallible human beings and not perfect angels, it follows that we constantly run the risk of infringing somebody's rules as to what constitutes proper behaviour. It is therefore nonsense to demand that people *should not*, or *must not* break your rules. By refusing to give others the right to be wrong, you are setting yourself up as a law-giver for everyone else you come in contact with. From that you can logically conclude that people who break your 'laws' are damnable souls who deserve no happiness and should be punished until they mend their ways. Also, it is absurd for you to believe 'I can't stand it when people treat me in such an irresponsible and unjust manner,' since you clearly do stand it. What you really mean is that you *will not*

*Dr Paul Hauck, *Calm Down* (Sheldon Press, 1980).

stand it, because what you say goes! Well, history shows us what happens when would-be gods get control and tell the rest of the world what they must and must not do!

Some other forms anger can take

Up to now, we have outlined a typical pattern of anger which, for obvious reasons, we term 'damning anger'. This kind of anger arises when the individual infers that some important goal has been frustrated, and/or that some person or institution has broken a personal rule of behaviour deemed important in the individual's personal domain. The anger arises, as we have seen, from the individual demanding that such frustration of his goals, or the transgression of an important rule of social or business behaviour, absolutely should not have happened; and because it did happen the person responsible deserves only condemnation for his or her bad deed. But what other forms does anger take?

Angry hurt

This type of anger arises when a person infers that he or she has been treated 'unfairly' and badly by some significant other, such as a spouse or love partner. Take the case of Nick and Sharon. After a year of marriage, during which time a planned vacation had been cancelled due to the demands of Nick's business, the couple decided to go away for a long weekend to a quiet country hotel. 'It'll be a second honeymoon, darling', said Nick to his wife. 'No interruptions from business partners, no phone calls, nothing to do with business; just the two of us alone!' Sharon felt delighted at the thought of having her husband to herself for several days and nights, especially after a year of spending long days and nights on her own when Nick had been attending meetings here and conferences there and sharing relatively little time with his wife.

On the morning of their departure, Nick received a phone call. He said: 'Look, darling, I can't explain now, but a really big deal has come up. The chance of a lifetime. I've got to take it. Be an angel and cancel the reservations for our trip. I'll make it up to you later!' Sharon felt very hurt and sobbed: 'Damn your bloody business! You are no good for treating me this way!' She stormed out of their flat and went to stay with a girlfriend.

Clearly, Sharon considered herself undeserving of such bad treatment. Her husband had promised her a second honeymoon and had broken that promise. She inferred that Nick had acted in an uncaring way towards her, that he thought more of his business than he did of her. In our previous example, we showed you the irrationality of condemning a person for acting in a way that would be considered unacceptable. While there may be an element of condemnation in Sharon's response to Nick's 'uncaring' behaviour, Sharon's main feeling of upset is one of 'hurt'. She feels hurt at being, as she sees it, reduced to playing second fiddle to Nick's business activities. Her irrational belief is quite clear: 'I do not deserve to be treated like this, and I must not get what I do not deserve.' She then concludes that Nick is a no good so-and-so for treating her as she did not deserve to be treated. Let's look at this notion of 'deserving' to see if the idea that life must give us what we deserve is sustainable in logic or in fact.

As generally used, it seems to mean that if you treat other people well, there is some rule of the universe that means they must treat you well in return. Or, if you have studied and worked hard and passed exams, then somehow some law or benevolent power will see to it that you must succeed in landing that job you were after. However, the facts of life are that there is no guarantee that if you are kind and considerate to others, they must respond kindly and considerately to you. They might, but then again they might not! And if you study conscientiously and work hard, you will, at best, improve your chances of succeeding in you chosen field. But it is not certain that you will. You may be struck down by some fatal illness, or the demand for your particular skills may no longer exist. Tough! That's the way life is, sometimes.

If you give up the idea that you must get what you think you deserve, and not get what you don't deserve, you will save yourself much needless unhappiness. This doesn't mean that whenever you are treated in what you consider an unfair manner, we are advising you to take it lying down. Far from it! If you give up the self-defeating belief that others must treat you as you think you deserve to be treated, and substitute the more rational: 'I prefer to be treated fairly (or not to be treated unfairly), but there is no reason why I *must* be treated in the way I prefer, and I do not *have* to get what I deserve', you will feel disappointed and sad, but not self-deprecating and hurt. You will be able to conclude: 'I'm not a non-entity because I am treated unfairly or inconsiderately; nor is the other person a rotter for acting inconsiderately, but only a fallible human being. I don't like his or her behaviour but everyone has a right to make mistakes. Now let me see what I can do to put my point of view and try to influence the other person to act in a "fairer" manner.' Your emotional consequence (C) following from those rational beliefs will be disappointment tinged with sadness and maybe annoyance. You will then be able to *act* constructively by communicating your feelings clearly, directly and assertively to the other person. In Sharon's case, she could inform Nick that while she appreciated the importance of his doing well in his business dealings, she also considered their own personal relationship to be more important, and that if he was not prepared to spend a reasonable amount of time with her in making their marriage a mutually satisfying, ongoing and caring relationship, she would consider leaving him. By contrast, if Sharon felt hurt by insisting that Nick *must* treat her with the consideration she 'deserved', she would tend to act aggressively and spitefully, or withdraw from him in such a way as to make their relationship even more difficult to mend.

Self-defensive or ego-defensive anger

This is the kind of anger you might experience in an encounter where you infer that the actions or responses of another person threaten your 'self-esteem'. When you feel angry, a typical response is retaliation against the other person or persons, usually in the form of a verbal attack, and followed often enough by withdrawing yourself from the other person's presence, as when you storm out of the house. Take, by way of illustration, an experience that one of the authors had a few years ago. A woman friend, whom he cared for a lot, accused him one evening of not being sufficiently concerned about her health after she had suffered an illness. She disparagingly compared his alleged lack of interest in her well-being with the concern solicitously expressed by all her other friends after her return from hospital. He made himself angry when she implied that his behaviour was evidence of a personal inadequacy. If he had acknowledged that she was right, he would have condemned himself for acting in a way he demanded he must never display. So his anger served as a cover for his self-denigration. He then foolishly 'blew his top' and hurled angry words at her, knowing that she would feel hurt by them. Then, slamming the door of her porch with a force which nearly detached it from its hinges, he stormed off into his car and drove home furious with rage. As if that was not stupid enough behaviour for one night, he felt guilty and extremely miserable as soon as his anger had died down and began savagely to curse himself for having acted as he did. He was sure he had blown the relationship for good this time. 'How could I have been so unbelievably stupid! How could I have done a rotten thing like that, and to *her* – of all people!' he repeated to himself over and over again. If you have read the previous chapter on guilt, you won't need any reminding of how very unhelpful and irrational such self-denigration can be. Anger doesn't just harm you directly; it also leads into other disturbed emotions and self-defeating behaviours that accompany them.

We have used the above illustration as an example of how *not* to react if ever you find yourself in a similar situation. Especially in close relationships, if your partner appears to be experiencing 'angry hurt' over something you are accused of having done or not done, the worst way to respond is to make counterallegations. It's like trying to dampen down a fire by throwing petrol on it. And saying you are sorry afterwards is unlikely to cut much ice, because in the heat of the moment you express your true feelings, and therefore your true thoughts. Saying 'I didn't mean it!' won't help, because at the time you really *did* mean it – and the other person knows it!

The episode described above is a good example of ego-defensive anger, and the guilt feelings that followed it clearly were generated by the self-denigration following the realization that a valued personal rule ('it is wrong to retaliate angrily against someone you love'), had been broken. The point we want you to pick up here is that the anger sprang, not from the friend's criticism, regardless of whether it was justified or not, but from the author's own low level of self-acceptance. Had he been more self-accepting on that occasion when being criticized for his lack of concern over his friend's health, he would have felt annoyed, but not angry. But he made himself angry to cover up his feelings of self-denigration when his woman friend pointed out to him a personal inadequacy. His anger resulted from the belief that she *must not* remind him of this personal inadequacy which he *must not* have and which would prove how rotten he was if he were to acknowledge its existence.

Self-rating, as we have been pointing out throughout this book, is not only untenable philosophically, but will lead you into many kinds of emotional difficulty. By contrast, self-acceptance is healthy and abets joyful living. When you accept yourself, you refuse to define yourself in terms of your achievements, or rate yourself according to what others think of you. Self-acceptance promotes tolerance of others, too, and thereby helps minimize intolerance and grandiosity, the roots of anger itself.

Truly accepting yourself, moreover, will help you give up most of your vulnerability, those feelings of hurt and self-pity which often fuel your anger, but it also encourages you to acknowledge your faults. In addition, losing your vulnerability will enable you to become more sensitive to others' opinions and feelings, and will help you to consider whether their criticisms of your behaviour are warranted or not.

An emotive technique for overcoming anger

Before we conclude our analysis of anger and how to deal with it, we would like to offer you a useful emotive technique which you can learn and use to help yourself overcome your propensity to anger. Known as

Rational-Emotive Imagery (REI), it was pioneered by Dr Maxie C. Maultsby, Jr, when he was chief psychiatrist at the University of Kentucky Medical Centre, and later modified and developed by Dr Albert Ellis, Executive Director of the Institute for Rational-Emotive Therapy in New York City. Here is what you do.

Think back in detail to a really angry confrontation you experienced personally. Picture yourself getting all steamed up. Feel yourself tensing up, ready to hurl angry words at your companion. Feel the hostility and allow yourself to feel distinctly uncomfortable as your anger builds up to a peak. Let yourself keenly experience your rage for a brief period of time. When you have actually felt your emotion for a while, push yourself as forcefully as you can to change the angry feeling in your gut so that instead you *only* feel very annoyed, and *not* furious and hostile, while still keeping the same scene vividly in your mind. If you find it difficult, keep persisting until you succeed. You have the ability to do it. So, concentrate, and do it! Now, when you have finally succeeded in pushing yourself to feel *only* very annoyed or irritated, look at what you did in your head to *make yourself* have these new, appropriate feelings. You will find that you have changed your belief system (point B), and in consequence, your feelings at point C. Look closely at what you told yourself to change your feelings from anger to annoyance. Once you see exactly what beliefs you have changed to make yourself feel appropriately annoyed rather than enraged, repeat the process. Make yourself feel angry; then make yourself feel displeased or annoyed. Then see exactly what beliefs you changed to change your feelings. Remember you create and control your feelings. They don't just suddenly appear out of nothing. Since you create your feelings you can also change them.

If you find this exercise difficult, keep practising it until you can do it. Keep working at it until you can easily change your upset feelings at point C to more appropriate feelings of displeasure or annoyance. Observe how you create and maintain your feelings at point B and become fully aware of exactly what you tell yourself to change your feelings about what was happening to you at point A, the activating event. Practise this REI procedure for at least ten minutes each day for the next few weeks. You can use REI not only to deal with your anger but also with anxiety, guilt and depression. The principle is the same in each case. With REI you change anxiety to concern, guilt to sorrow or remorse, depression to sadness or disappointment. If you conscientiously practise this kind of REI you will find that whenever you experience some disturbed emotion, you will tend automatically to feel some form of rational displeasure rather than some emotional upset.

Some people find mental imagery more difficult than others. For those who do, and for those of you who tend to avoid doing the exercises but would welcome encouragement to carry them out, we recommend that you use the self-management methods we outlined in Chapter 2 of this book. These methods will help you get going. Once you make a start you will tend to find it easier to continue doing your REI practice. When you see the results you get from it, you may even come to look forward to it. So, go ahead and practise!

Conclusion

In this chapter, we have tried to show you in various ways how to recognize, challenge and eliminate the anger that can frustrate your goals and damage your personal and interpersonal relationships. The personal and social cost of anger is enormous. Anger, and the low frustration tolerance which fuels it, is often a direct cause of murder, and an important contributory cause of child abuse and of both individual and mob violence. Anger is a direct cause of many a breakdown of marriage and other close relationships which would otherwise have survived quite happily. Anger can be a killer in the literal sense; it can trigger off a heart attack in those with cardio-vascular problems.

Frustrations are an everyday experience for most of us. If we didn't have strong desires to achieve our aims and to get what we want from life, frustration of our wishes would not be a problem. But if we had no desire, it is unlikely we would survive, individually, or as a species. When our desires are blocked, momentarily or for longer periods, it is natural to feel annoyance or displeasure. Our displeasure motivates us to act assertively to remove the sources obstructing the realization of our wishes. In that sense it is healthy and rational because it promotes our survival and the achievement of future pleasure. The trouble begins when we escalate our legitimate desires, wishes or preferences into dictatorial commands that our will be done. Anger stems from being demanding, from grandiosity, from playing the two-year-old. Anger may occasionally enable you to get your way when others are too scared to resist your demands. But not for long! Sooner or later, it will do you in.

We cannot control how other people think and feel, but we can control – and change – how *we* think and feel. You have now been given the tools – a set of effective techniques – to home in on your anger-creating beliefs and to uproot and replace them with sensible life-enhancing philosophies. As adult humans, we have the capability to think and act sanely. If you study and use the methods we have spelled out in this book to overcome your tendency to upset yourself emotionally, you can help to create a saner and safer world for yourself and your loved ones to live in.

SUMMARY POINTS FOR CHAPTER 5

(1) Annoyance, irritation and displeasure are not the same thing as anger. Feelings of annoyance in response to a situation where your wishes are blocked or your aims frustrated, can be healthy because disliking some situation can motivate you to act assertively to change it. Annoyance, displeasure and irritation with people and situations which block you in the pursuit of your aims, is a normal part of living.

(2) Anger is not only a powerful feeling of antipathy directed towards other people but can also have damaging physiological side-effects on the person who is angry.

(3) Most people appear to believe that their anger is caused by other people or by external happenings outside their control. Thus, believing that feelings of anger are stirred up by outside forces, various palliative measures are proposed by some people to release these feelings – activities recommended include pillow-punching, freely expressing your anger towards someone by mutual arrangement, or just being placid. None of these measures work very well because they fail to get to the root of the problem of anger.

(4) The RET approach to the problem of anger is the same approach as we have used in dealing with anxiety, guilt and depression. The sources of anger are located in your belief system, that cluster of beliefs concerning how you think the world *should* be, but usually isn't!

(5) The first step is to identify your own anger-creating philosophies by using the A-B-C framework and then to challenge and dispute the irrational belief components in your anger-generating philosophies until you extirpate them and replace them with more rational and helpful ideas and attitudes.

(6) Generally speaking, when you are frustrated and/or inconvenienced or treated in a manner you consider 'unfair', you may react angrily to the person or situation concerned. However, your anger springs not from the activating event or circumstance but from your dictatorial command that you *must not* be treated in an 'unfair' manner, and that when you are treated as you think you must not be, it's awful, and you can't stand it, and whoever is responsible must be punished because he or she deserves to be punished.

(7) These irrational ideas lie at the core of your anger. They create and sustain it. However, when you apply rational analysis to these beliefs, they turn out to be logically absurd and indefensible.

(8) In addition to the methods set out to help you change your thinking about anger, self-defeating and other emotional states such as anxiety and guilt, we introduced a form of emotional re-education which we termed Rational-Emotive Imagery (REI). If you conscientiously practise REI in conjunction with the methods of logical and scientific analysis of your irrational beliefs which we demonstrated in detail, you will find it harder to become angry in future. In time, if you work at using RET until it becomes a habit, you will rarely anger yourself over practically anything. If a saner, calmer more enjoyable life is what you want, ridding yourself of anger is an important step towards your goal.

6

Love Problems

Probably no subject has attracted more attention in modern times than love. More books have been written, more songs have been sung, more sermons have been preached about love than about any other subject. Perhaps it is hardly surprising, then, in view of this outpouring of human energy and devotion to Eros, that love, or the lack of it, is frequently seen as a major problem in the lives of literally millions of people all over the world. The many column inches of space in popular newspapers and magazines devoted to answering readers' questions on love and related matters, and to giving advice to the love-lorn, surely testify to an apparently universal preoccupation with the subject of love, and a seemingly insatiable appetite for it.

But what is love? There is romantic love, and conjugal love, childhood love, motherly love, and cupboard love. We've even heard of platonic love. Rather than attempt to supply a definition which would encompass this breathtaking variety of love, we prefer to offer you some unusual – and, we hope, useful – RET insights into the real nature of some problems commonly associated with love. As we proceed, you may come to realize that we, too, have our own ideas as to what love 'is'.

Meanwhile, we will begin by taking a brief look at some popular myths about love. Then we shall pick up the ideas underlying one or two of these myths to show you that, regardless of the kind of emotional problem you may experience with regard to love, or the loss of it, by itself love cannot be the direct cause of that problem. Since the system of counselling we espouse is largely a theory of, as well as a practical approach to, interpersonal relationships, we consider it is particularly well suited to dealing with love problems and their treatment.

Some popular myths about love

Here are just a few of the more popular myths about love, especially romantic love, in our Western culture:

(1) You can love truly only one person at any one time.
(2) Unless you become extremely jealous when someone you love goes off with some other person, that proves that you did not really love that person in the first place.
(3) It is terrible to be rejected by someone for whom you have a deep

81

romantic love, and you must feel so upset that only after you have experienced a long period of grief and depression can you get your 'heart high enough' to go out and look for someone else to fall in love with again.

We could list many more myths surrounding love, sex and marriage. You can hear many of them reaffirmed almost daily in popular music lyrics, from Sinatra to Madonna and Michael Jackson. Personally, we like some of the music, but, oh, those lyrics! When you add to these myths such widespread irrational ideas as the idea that adult human beings have a deep *need* for love, and that getting it is a dire necessity, it is clear that counsellors will seldom, if ever, be out of work.

Let's pick up now on one of the above-mentioned myths about love –the idea that it is terrible to be rejected by your lover and that you must go through a long period of mourning before you can, with great difficulty, fall in love again with someone else.

When rejection is a problem

Rejection may occur at the beginning of a relationship when a partner changes his or her mind about getting involved. More troubling, perhaps, is the case where a love relationship has been established with a chosen partner on a reciprocal basis, and after a time one of them suddenly breaks off the relationship, sometimes without giving the other partner any explanation whatsoever. In most such cases, the emotional problem resulting from the loss which the rejected partner suffers may be recognized as depression, hurt, anxiety, anger or even guilt. The behavioural consequences of these disturbed emotions occasionally make the newspaper headlines as when the outcome is a spectacular suicide or a murder. As RET counsellors dedicated to helping people to survive as happily as possible, we deplore the loss of life which sometimes occurs in those circumstances. To us, this loss of life is tragic and unnecessary. Moreover, if you believe, as we do, that this life is the only chance you have of life on earth, it follows that too much time spent in self-pity following a rejection is time wasted which could be put to better use – for example, going out and finding a new love partner, or becoming creatively absorbed in some long-range project that is important to you. For these reasons, we try to help people suffering a loss of love to overcome their distress in as quick and efficient a manner as possible. The following example will show you how we go about it.

A case of rejection

Maureen, a 37-year-old teacher, had been separated from her husband for a year when she met Martin, an accountant, 41 years old and divorced. It wasn't exactly love at first sight, but Martin, who had known her for several years before they got together, confessed to 'always having had a crush on Maureen'. When they finally got together one weekend, Martin was over the moon. Their relationship quickly blossomed and things seemed to be going well during the months following their meeting.

Then, one evening on their way home from a trip up to town, Maureen, who had been unusually silent throughout the journey home in Martin's car, told Martin as he saw her to the door of her flat that their relationship was over, and bid him goodnight. Martin returned to his home in a daze, unable to believe what had happened to him. Within a few days, Martin developed a deep depression. For months Martin anguished over what had caused his lover to leave him so unexpectedly. 'If only she had told me *why!*' Martin exclaimed. 'I'm not saying she hadn't the right to break off the relationship, although that was hard enough to take after all she had come to mean to me. I loved that girl! But it was the *way* she did it; just to finish it like that (snapping his fingers), without even a word of explanation, not even a minute of discussion – *that's* what really hurt! If only she had told me why she wanted to go, I could have accepted it. We could have discussed her reasons. But she didn't.even give me any, she just stopped seeing me, just like that! It made me feel awful; in fact I've never felt so miserable in all my entire life. I kept asking myself, "What could I have done, or said to make her do a thing like that to me. But she never once told me, and ignored all my letters asking her for an explanation." '

Putting Martin's experience in terms of our A-B-C model, we endeavoured to teach him that it was not the fact that his girlfriend had rejected him at point A which made him desperately 'hurt' or depressed at point C. Rather, it was the nonsensical things that he told himself at point B *about* what happened to him at point A. As we proceed to uncover the irrational beliefs which created Martin's depression, you will, we hope, appreciate that the aim of the counselling process is to enable Martin to learn that there is nothing to be afraid of in being rejected or spurned by another, and that his 'hurt' or depression at being rejected is nothing more than an irrational idea in his own head, an unsustainable assumption that he unthinkingly perpetuates by constant repetition. So, look closely now at what Martin was telling himself at point B to produce his feelings of hurt and depression. When you have done so, and appreciated why Martin's beliefs about rejection are invalid, we will suggest what rational alternative views he could take about his situation. Martin's beliefs about being rejected by Maureen, and specifically about the way it happened, were the following:

(1) 'I *should not* have been rejected, especially in the inconsiderate way it happened, because that proves there was something radically wrong with me. And so I couldn't have been worthy of her to start with. Now I'll probably never find another fine person like her no matter how hard I try.'

(2) 'If I was really attractive and competent, this would never have happened. This rejection, as well as my previous divorce, proves I really am no good at winning and keeping the love of a woman I truly care about.'

(3) 'I can't stand Maureen thinking badly of me! I must have struck her as a right useless person when she didn't even tell me why she was leaving me.'

(4) 'I'm never going to take the risk of being treated like that again!'

(5) 'I'll never meet anyone like Maureen who will accept me and make up for the kind of relationship I had with her in the beginning. And if I can't be happy at all, what's the point of going on living?'

Since Martin tenaciously clung to these beliefs he had a difficult time in overcoming his severely depressed mood. He refused to look for other acceptable love partners, and became so obsessed with the loss of his partner that his business and social life suffered. His friends drifted away as he became more miserable, and Martin took their loss of interest in him as 'proof' that he really was an incompetent idiot who would never enjoy an intimate relationship with anyone else.

As is usual in RET counselling, these irrational beliefs and unsupportable inferences were logically examined and challenged. Let's take them one by one.

Where is the evidence for Martin's belief that 'I *should not* have been rejected?' If you're rejected, you're rejected. Tough! There is no law which says you should not be rejected. If there was such a law, then you would not be rejected. When you demand that something should, or should not, be the case, you are really issuing a command that the world must be the way you want it to be. Since none of us has the power to make the world accord us our wishes, we had better realistically accept our limitations in this respect and give up our 'shoulds' and 'musts' about the universe.

Next, Martin upset himself over what he considered Maureen's inconsiderate behaviour in not giving him her reasons for breaking off their relationship. Now, this was only an inference on Martin's part, as was also his conviction that there must have been something radically wrong with him. It is possible that Maureen chose not to give Martin her reasons because she thought it was kinder for her not to tell him, that a quick clean break was better than lengthy explanations. She could, therefore, have been acting quite considerately. But because Martin had a low level of self-acceptance, it did not occur to him that her silence might have been motivated out of consideration for his feelings, as opposed to her own. He easily assumed, because of his pronounced self-deprecating tendencies, that *he* must be at fault and that Maureen had perceived his weaknesses. In fact, it is possible that Maureen could have decided to end their affair for reasons of her own, quite unconnected with Martin's self-alleged shortcomings. However, let's assume that Maureen did act inconsiderately. It is often a good idea to show people that even if their worst fears about what has happened to them are true, the rejection, or whatever they are upset about, is still only an inconvenience, and not a truly terrible thing. And, for good measure, let us also assume that Maureen rejected Martin for having a fault which many other women would also have rejected him for. Let's suppose that Martin invariably thought he was right about everything and that other people, including Maureen, were mostly wrong. This might well explain why Maureen broke off their relationship in the way that she did!

First, note that Martin does not deny that Maureen had the right to break off the relationship. What he does appear to deny is Maureen's right to leave him without discussing her reasons for doing so. He is, in effect, telling himself: 'When a woman friend leaves me, she must give me an explanation!' Apart from being illogical, where is the evidence that Maureen must give him an explanation for her decision to break off with him? If Martin could grant that Maureen had the right to sever their relationship, should he not logically have accepted that she also had the right to break away without having to explain her reasons to him? Whether or not it would have been better had Maureen explained her reasons before leaving is beside the point. The real issue is whether Maureen was obliged to tell Martin why she had decided to leave him. Or more generally, whether it is rational to demand that other people give us an explanation, or apology, for *anything* they do? Granted, it would be better if others sometimes explained to us why they acted the way they did, and made suitable apologies for inconsiderate behaviour towards us. But where is it written that they *must* do so?

Martin was upset because he irrationally believed, as millions of people do, that other people must treat him fairly and considerately, and that it is horrible when they don't. If you demand that other people must treat you fairly and considerately, and kindly offer you reasons for their behaviour, you are going to be frequently disappointed! There is no harm in asking for an explanation when you are put to some trouble or inconvenience; and quite often calmly and assertively standing up for your rights will earn you others' respect. But demanding that others give you what you think they owe you is self-defeating and likely to get you nowhere.

Martin's next error was to assume that the manner in which Maureen broke off the relationship proved that there was something 'radically wrong' with him. But our assumption was that the relationship was terminated because Maureen found Martin's intolerance of other people's opinions objectionable, and unacceptable to her. Does that prove that there was something radically wrong with him? No! All it proves is that Martin had a particular trait – his intolerance of other people's opinions – which Maureen, and probably most women, would have found obnoxious and unacceptable. But an obnoxious trait does not make you an obnoxious person. As we have pointed out in previous chapters, a person is not the same thing as his or her traits or actions. You cannot legitimately rate a person. You can only give their behaviour, their personal characteristics, a rating in terms of some value system. A person may have a certain extrinsic value to others depending upon what he or she does. But a person's *intrinsic* value, or your value to yourself, is not measurable by any external standards. Thus, if Martin had an unfortunate characteristic, his intolerance, he could still accept himself with his failing, and once he recognized it as such, he could work to rid himself of it in the interests of winning a good relationship later with some other woman. In RET counselling, we do not condemn the person for having an undesirable aspect to his character, instead we accept the individual unconditionally and encourage him to view himself in a less self-condemning manner as a prelude to working towards changing unhelpful characteristics and behaviours.

Now we come to Martin's belief that if he was 'really attractive and competent, this would never have happened'. This is an unwarrantable assumption. Is it true that people who are attractive and act competently *never* get rejected? Obviously not! Rejection may occur less often if you are attractive and behave competently, but it is by no means ruled out completely. Martin then goes on to compare his rejection with his divorce and concludes that his double failure proves that he is really no good at winning or keeping the love of a woman he really cares about. This is a good example of over-generalization. How do his two failures in the dating and mating game prove that he is no good at all? All his previous failures prove is that he failed on these occasions to maintain an ongoing relationship. His failures don't make *him* a failure, nor do they imply that he can never succeed in future in creating and maintaining a good relationship with someone else. Moreover, Martin's self-deprecating 'I am no good at keeping a relationship going' will do nothing to help him look at his own attitudes and values and discover how he could change his self-defeating outlook and replace it with more sensible views on relating well to others.

We now move on to Martin's belief that he *can't stand* Maureen thinking badly of him. He clearly pities himself for having been treated so 'unfairly' and the 'dreadful' part of it was that she did not choose to explain why she was leaving, as he thought she *must!* 'She *must* give me an explanation!' is the irrational idea here which upset Martin. As we have shown above, the world doesn't *have to* owe you fair play, or indeed, anything.

Martin's determination 'never to risk being treated like that again' also sprang from his low level of self-acceptance and his low level of frustration tolerance. Martin was shown that if he never took any risks of rejection and simply sat on his rump feeling sorry for himself, then he most probably would not find himself a future partner more suited to him. Life itself is a risk. There are no guarantees in the universe. Martin came to see that if he never overcame his irrational fears of risking rejection, he was practically ensuring he would remain permanently without the kind of relationship he claimed he wanted.

Martin's next conviction that he would never be accepted by anyone who could compare with Maureen is yet another example of an unfounded assumption and over-generalization. Certainly, if Martin never risked going out and looking for a possible replacement for Maureen, because he feared rejection, he would be most unlikely to wind up with anyone. Also, so long as Martin considered himself 'unworthy' of winning a relationship comparable to the one he had lost, this would almost guarantee he would be unsuccessful because potential partners would see what a negative view he had of himself, and would tend to turn away from him. A point to bear in mind here is that people will tend to shy away from you if they sense that you are vulnerable to the possibility of rejection.

As Martin worked on the beliefs underlying his low opinion of himself, he began to see that he was not the same thing as his acts. He realized that his good deeds and performances did not make him a good person any more than his failures and mistaken acts made him a bad person, but merely a person with some good traits and some poor traits who occasionally acted well and competently and at other times less well and incompetently. As Martin began to truly accept himself and ceased condemning himself for his failures he was able to take a more rational view of losing his love relationship with Maureen. He now was able to convince himself that: 'It's too bad that Maureeen rejected me, and I wish she hadn't; but that's the way things are. Tough! Maybe I'll try to contact her again next week, after all I've nothing to lose. If she tells me there's absolutely no way we're going to get back together again, or even if she refuses to talk to me, tough again! It's not the end of the world. I won't like it, but I definitely can stand it. If she doesn't want to resume our relationship, I'll look for someone else. Even if I get rejected by the next ninety-nine women, there's always the hundredth.'

As you can see from Martin's last remark, he had made a fundamental change in his attitude towards the possibility of finding himself a suitable partner. He not only changed his earlier irrational views on the intellectual level, but had so thoroughly convinced himself of the truth of the more rational ideas he had acquired that he was prepared to *act* on them, to *risk* becoming emotionally involved with other possible partners with the ever-present possibility of being rejected by them.

An important gain from his counselling was Martin's ability to accept himself unconditionally. He was able to look back on his previous relationship with Maureen and admit that she had been a fine partner for him, but also to accept that there would be other women in his life with whom he could have an equally good or even better relationship. Instead of condemning his former partner for treating him inconsiderately, he could truthfully say, and believe: 'The woman whose love I lost meant a great deal to me, but she had her own reasons for leaving me. It is possible that these reasons may have had relatively little to do with me as a person, or with the ways in which I behaved during our friendship. But it is more likely that she found some of my behaviour unacceptable. I admit that I am intolerant of views with which I disagree, and when I disagreed with her, I frequently did so in a manner which she considered brusque and dismissive. But now that I am aware of my shortcomings and fully acknowledge them, I will do my best to change my attitudes and to behave in a more constructive and helpful manner in future.' Thus, Martin began to rethink his former failure to maintain an ongoing relationship with Maureen, as well with as his ex-wife, and to see his failures as a challenge to be met and learned from, rather than a horror to be depressed about. In this type of counselling, we aim to help the client secure a fundamental restructuring of his or her basic philosophy rather than to be content with helping the client feel better about the particular problem presented for discussion. To the extent that the client achieves this goal, it is likely that he or she will become only minimally emotionally upset by any problem encountered in future.

The main points we would like you to learn from this demonstration are the following. First, when you are rejected by someone whose love or approval you care about winning and retaining, admit that this is annoying and frustrating, but refrain from convincing yourself that it is horrible and that you can't stand it. It is especially important to remember that being rejected cannot prove anything about your self-worth, or value to yourself. Suppose it really is your fault that you are rejected. It often will not be your fault – your partner may leave you for reasons quite unconnected with you or the quality of your contribution to your relationship; but suppose it is, at least partly, your fault. Being a fallible, error-prone human being, you can logically conclude that you will make many errors throughout your life, and will therefore often be rejected by people whose approval you would strongly prefer to retain. But being rejected does not make you a rejectee! Get hold of that idea, think about it, and repeat it to yourself many times until you see that it is true. Then, the next time somebody turns you down, instead of putting yourself down, fully accept yourself in spite of the other person's disapproval and try to see how you can improve your chances by making fewer errors in future and increasing the probability of being accepted by someone else.

Second, do not try to eradicate your desire for love or approval. To desire strongly to succeed in love is rational and healthy. Eliminate only your dire, all-consuming love *needs*.

Adults don't need love

The notion that we all *need* love is still widely held. Popular music, of both yesterday's and today's variety, still plugs the idea that we are nothing without love. If that were true, we'd all be dead by now! Even some psychologists still assert that we need love. OK, babies and young children obviously need love. Unless there was someone around to succour and care for them, they would simply die of neglect. Children *literally* depend on others, especially their parents, to find food, clothing, shelter and medical care, if they are to thrive and be happy. We are all saddened and appalled whenever we read or hear of children suffering or even dying through mistreatment and neglect by those adults charged with their care. But we are not children.

Strictly speaking, to say we need something is to claim that we would die without it. The only things we need to survive are food and water, shelter and air. Everything else is optional. Of course, we tend to feel good when we are loved or admired by significant others, and we would feel much less happy if we *never* received any love or approval from others. But *wanting* something and *needing* it are two entirely different things. If you believe that adult humans *need* love and approval, and that they cannot live happily without it, we invite you to consider these alternative beliefs:

(1) If you *always* need love, you are going to have to appear lovable, especially to those whose love you desperately 'need'. Do you know anybody who has been lovable right throughout his or her entire life? Perhaps you are lovable today, meaning that you have certain traits or personality characteristics, etc., which some other people find lovable? But can you guarantee that you will still be lovable tomorrow?

(2) If you demand love from certain people around you, you are unlikely to get it from all of them. Some may disapprove of you because you happen to lack some quality they deem important, or possess some quality they find abhorrent. You may be too short in height, or too thin, or have the 'wrong' colour of skin, or speak with too high-pitched a voice. You can do practically nothing about these in-born characteristics. Others will disapprove of you all your life because they don't trust you due to some mistake you made in your initial encounter with them. Still others will be more interested in getting *you* to love *them*!

(3) Once you get the love you think you need, you will tend to worry about how long it is going to last, and whether or not the other person loves you enough. If your anxiety becomes obvious enough, the other person may well begin to feel put off by your continual need for reassurance.

(4) We have found sometimes that individuals with a dire need for love and approval tend to become compulsive attention-seekers, forever seeking popularity by trying to appear witty and great company to anyone who can be persuaded to listen. When this doesn't work (as after a while it doesn't), the individual adopts a self-pitying attitude and complains of being ignored. All this 'song and dance' act is mostly a cover-up for underlying feelings of worthlessness. In effect, this individual is saying: 'I must have your love or be thought highly of, because I remain a rotten individual who cannot manage my own life by myself. Therefore I *need* your love and your approval.' The more you cover up your underlying feelings of worthlessness, the less likely are you to tackle them and learn to stand on your own feet and manage your own life with, or without, other people's approval.

(5) One more point you might consider is the cost to you in surrendering your own wishes when you ceaselessly strive to win love or approval from selected individuals. The more you go out of your way to buy others' approval – by, for example, always being

the ever-present helpmate, putting others' wishes before your own, and generally playing the role of a doormat – you will wind up living your life doing what others want you to do, rather than striving for your own goals and values. Lots of people will happily allow you to cater to their every whim or wish, but you will find that ultimately they will lose respect for you, and cease to care for you. Your incessant attentions may even bore and annoy them so that they eventually come to despise you. Thus, you could lose out on two counts when you have an inordinate need for love or approval.

How to maximize your chances of winning love

What can you rationally do to win the love of someone you care for? First of all, learn to accept yourself, regardless of whether certain significant others love you or not. Why is it irrational to make your self-acceptance conditional upon winning the love or approval of others? If you can only accept yourself as a human being with intrinsic worth or value to yourself when significant others confer upon you their seal of approval, you are demanding a guarantee of acceptability before you can accept yourself. How could anyone get a guarantee of acceptability? Guarantees don't exist. If you demand a guarantee, you are going to be miserable all your life; you will be miserable not only when you are not accepted (because that 'proves' that you are no good), but also when you are accepted; for if you are accepted today, you are going to worry about being accepted tomorrow, and the next day, and the next!

Not only are you going to feel anxious, but in seeking love to raise your 'self-esteem' you are in effect saying: 'I am only worthwhile when someone loves me.' Since there will be times when you may find nobody to love you, your so-called self-esteem will take a nosedive and your life will be experienced as a roller-coaster in which you feel good when you have love, and miserable when you don't.

Once you realize that true self-respect – or self-acceptance (which we consider a better term because it avoids implying any degree of self-rating) – never comes from the approval of others, but from a decision to accept yourself as a fallible human being who cannot be given a single rating, and from pursuing your own interests whether or not others approve of your activities, you will find that *loving* can be an absorbing, creative and growth-enhancing occupation, whether or not you are loved in return.

Second, try to win the approval of significant others for practical reasons, such as companionship, conversational ability, or some kind of artistic achievement or accomplishment which can give pleasure to

91

yourself and others. You are not loved for *yourself*, but for your qualities of mind and character, your characteristics, traits, abilities or appearance. You may be loved because you are kind and caring, or for your strength and courage, or for literally scores of different reasons. When someone sees in you the embodiment of his or her deepest desires and aspirations, that person will readily feel loving towards you. Being loved has many advantages. So long as you choose to live in a social group, wanting acceptance, approval and some degree of care from the members of your social group is sane and healthy. We do not go along with the Zen Buddhist view that you should give up all desire for earthly satisfactions. Instead, we support the human desire to love and be loved, but we do not view it as an absolute necessity.

Third, concentrate on giving love rather than receiving it. 'Love begets love', as the saying goes. It doesn't always work out like that, of course, but it often does. If you seek to live fully and vitally, then actively devote yourself to various people, things and ideas outside yourself, but do so without sacrificing yourself. The feeling of being alive doesn't come from passively accepting whatever life offers you, but from doing, looking and reaching outwards. You will find that when you give up worrying self-centredly about being loved enough, you will more easily become involved in outside interests and activities and more motivated to follow enthusiastically your own basic bents and to devote yourself to activities that you consider personally enjoyable and satisfying from a long-term perspective.

Above all, don't confuse getting love or approval from others with your personal worth or value to yourself. No matter how much others may love you or value you for their own benefit, they cannot, by loving you, give you intrinsic worth or value to yourself. If you can really accept this important truth – that you need never rate your *self*, your essence, in any way whatsoever, you will tend to lose your desperate need for others' approval. Once your dire need for their acceptance evaporates, you will readily enjoy the practical advantages stemming from others' approval, but no longer foolishly define your worth as a human in terms of receiving or not receiving their love or approval.

Jealousy

Jealousy, the green-eyed monster, can be as damaging to your health and to your relationships as that other great disrupter of happiness – anger. In the previous chapter, we showed you why anger is a destroyer of human life and happiness and what you can do to minimize your propensity to anger. In this section we shall look at how jealousy arises and show you how you can achieve a more happy existence by ridding yourself of jealousy or helping someone you know who suffers from jealousy. We use the word 'suffer' advisedly. For it isn't just the jealous person who suffers from the obsessive fear and sick feeling inside with which he or she contends: the person who is the victim of jealousy suffers, and there is a ripple effect which can affect people only remotely connected with the jealous individual. One of the authors of this book had the experience some years ago of being the victim of a jealous woman because he happened to know her friend rather too well for this jealous woman's liking. She did her best to disrupt his friendship with this other woman, and although he discovered later that this jealous woman was psychotic, and had narrowly escaped being placed in an institution, that hardly made her machinations and meddling any easier to tolerate. The jealous person is possessive and dictatorial to a degree which makes living with such a person a real pain in the neck. If you have a problem with jealousy, either in relation to yourself, or with some other person such as a friend or relative, you will find it helpful to acquire some RET insights into the nature of jealousy and how to reduce or eliminate it.

The A-B-C of jealousy

There are really two forms of jealousy and it is important to distinguish the one from the other. There is rational jealousy, and there is irrational jealousy. It is unfortunate that the English language does not appear to possess a separate word to denote rational jealousy. In the previous chapter, we were able to make a distinction between (irrational) anger and (rational) annoyance. But with jealousy we have to make do with the one word.

Take rational jealousy first. If you desire to maintain an ongoing relationship with someone you love, and you become concerned about the relationship being disrupted due to your beloved paying a lot of attention to someone else, you can be rationally jealous. Why? Because there is a possibility of your being deprived of your partner's presence and companionship, or even of losing him or her altogether. Since you would obviously be able to prove you would be deprived in various ways if your partner did leave you for someone else, you can hardly be expected to like the situation. Thus, you could legitimately claim to feel frustrated by your loss and disappointed at not being able to participate in further intimate sharing of your life with your partner, but you would not be severely disturbed about it.

Now contrast the above state of affairs with what happens when you are irrationally jealous. As with rational jealousy, you may believe there is a possibility of losing your partner. But the emotional consequences for you, at point C, may include serious anxiety, anger or depression. You obsessively speculate about where your partner is, what he or she is doing and who he or she is with. You look for signs of infidelity, try to listen to your partner's phone calls, and even have him or her followed in the hope of uncovering some compromising situation. This state of mind typically stems from a number of irrational beliefs, at point B, such as the following:

(1) 'I must have a guarantee that my partner is interested only in me and will continue to love me indefinitely.'
(2) 'If my partner doesn't make me the sole interest and object of his or her love, that would be awful and I couldn't stand it.'
(3) 'If my partner leaves me or even becomes interested in someone else, that proves that I am no good.'
(4) 'If my partner leaves me or even becomes interested in someone else, that proves that he (and/or the other person) is no good.'

If you recall what we pointed out in our remarks about rejection, you will easily recognize the irrationality of the first of these statements. There simply are no guarantees in the world. How can anyone *guarantee* to love you indefinitely? As we said before, if you must have guarantees, you are on a hiding to nothing. You will be miserable if you get them and miserable if you don't. Go back and read what we wrote about guarantees in the section on rejection if you have forgotten that important point.

Now look at the second irrational statement. You are saying here that, unless your partner makes you the linchpin of his or her life and refuses to have anything to do with anyone else, you couldn't stand it and it would be awful. Ask yourself: does this make sense? You obviously can stand anything until you die. Is it realistic to demand eternal devotion from someone? Realistically, you may strive to create and maintain a good exclusive loving relationship with your partner so that he or she would be unlikely to want anything different, and would be perfectly happy with you. But how likely are you to get your ideal relationship by *demanding* it? Very unlikely, we would say!

Similarly with the third irrational statement. Can you recognize here the presence of a low level of self-acceptance? 'Unless I am accepted by my partner (which would be proved by his or her never leaving me for anyone else) I cannot accept myself.' We have already shown you that you should preferably accept yourself unconditionally and that if you make accepting yourself conditional upon what someone else thinks of you, your goose is cooked. Self-acceptance, as we have been emphasizing throughout this book, is one of the most valuable assets you can achieve. Since the lack of it is one of the root causes of irrational jealousy, it follows that if you can acquire true unconditional self-acceptance, you will find it difficult to become irrationally jealous of anyone.

The fourth irrational statement is an example of 'angry hurt' which we discussed in the previous chapter. Since neither anger nor jealousy will do you or your love relationships any good, what changes would you make in your ideas to ensure that in the event of a possible loss of love, you would feel only rationally jealous, and not allow yourself to stray into the quicksand of irrational jealousy? We suggest the following alternative ideas would enable you to stay rationally jealous, rather than become severely upset in the event of a withdrawal of your partner in favour of some other person:

(1) 'I would certainly like you to stay and care only for me, but there is no reason why you have to do so. I can still be happy without you, although not as happy as I could be if you were to remain with me.'

(2) 'I love you dearly and want no one else, but you are not obliged on that account to love me in return, or to feel that you must restrict your love interest to me alone. I would certainly prefer you to, but you don't have to.'

(3) 'If you leave me or become interested in someone else, I would definitely not like that. But I will accept myself unconditionally if these things happen.'

(4) 'If you treat me unfairly or inconsiderately, I shall not condemn you for your poor behaviour, although I shall not like it. Instead, I shall try to understand your feelings and motivations and see if I can't persuade you to be more loving towards me.'

If you think along these lines, you will save yourself much needless emotional turmoil. If you and your partner see no great advantages to separating and, if you are married, divorcing, you might be able to negotiate some new arrangement in which you both agree to a more open relationship or some form of non-monogamous arrangement. Rational jealousy can enable you to avoid the destruction of a relationship you might both wish to retain, and can help keep alive certain aspects of it which you both agree are of value to you. By contrast, becoming irrationally jealous of your partner will almost certainly create a degree of emotional misery for yourself, and probably for your partner as well. The end result could be the destruction of your relationship with your partner, with nothing worthwhile left to show for it.

What to look for in a partner

Let's assume that you are not desperately seeking love, that you are fairly happy with your life, but that you would very much like to have a good, sound loving relationship with a member of the opposite sex. Let's also assume that you are a woman who is seeking a desirable partner, although most of what we are going to say can apply to men as well.

In no sense are we about to issue you with a set of definitive guidelines on how to look, where to look, or what to do with the woman or man who seems to be the answer to your prayers. To accomplish that in any adequate way would justify a book in itself. Instead, we hope to offer you some advice, which, if it doesn't exactly net you the man (or woman) of your dreams, may at least help you to avoid getting entangled with some of the more *un*suitable characters around with whom you may come in contact.

What sort of attributes would we suggest that you look for in a potential long-term or marriage partner?

Compatibility

In the heyday of the romantic novel, romantic love was held to be all important. Boy meets girl and they fall in love. Once they felt sure they were in love, the couple were expected to proceed to the altar. The revolution in people's lifestyles produced by twentieth-century developments in science, technology and medicine brought about changing attitudes to love, marriage and divorce. The pendulum swung the other way, and we began to hear a lot about 'compatibility' and less about 'love' as the guarantor of happy relationships. Our own view is that there are no guarantees of anything, except death – and scientists are even now working on that! We are not knocking romantic love – or any other kind of love. It is how you experience it that matters. But let's see what we mean by 'compatibility', without assuming that it is necessarily more important than love, or any other component of a successful relationship.

First, love and compatibility are not the same thing. You can love someone dearly but be quite incompatible living partners. Your tastes and interests can differ. There will seldom, if ever, be complete harmony between two people on matters of taste, interests and personal habits. The important question is how *much* your tastes and interests differ. You are not necessarily wrong because you are different. You may be tidy and like to keep your home clean, while your partner is sloppy and never puts anything away. You may enjoy extended conversations on a wide range of subjects, while your partner likes nothing better than to spend several nights a week with his buddies round at the local. Or he may be an armchair sports fanatic and spend much of his time glued to the TV, leaving you to make the meals, keep the house clean and do the shopping. Some of these incompatibilities can be minimized by negotiating compromises in a spirit of goodwill. Thus, if he will agree to take you to the opera once a month, you will let him go to his football match with his friends. Some things, however, may not be negotiable. For example, if you detest smoking, and your potential partner chain-smokes cigarettes, you would be wise to rule him out as a long-term prospect. Know what your deepest desires and values are. If you happen to be a staunch Christian, for example, you would be unwise to consider linking up with an equally convinced atheist, no matter how attractive your atheist friend may be to you in other ways. Stick to your guns, and get to know your potential partner as well as possible *before* you decide to settle down for the fifty or so years that possibly lie ahead. If you discover some basic incompatibility between you, regretfully but firmly eliminate that person from your list of possible partners, no matter how madly attached you may already have become to him. Remember, you have to live with your choices!

Get to know your suitor's family and friends. They will often reveal things about your would-be lover that he has never mentioned to you. And because we are all moulded to some degree by our family and friendship associations, getting to know his family's traits and habits, especially their less endearing ones, will give you a good idea of what to expect from him should you decide to settle down with him. Be romantic, if you will, but keep your feet on the ground!

Emotional stability

One of the greatest blocks to getting along well with someone in a close relationship is emotional disturbance. If you or your potential partner have a short temper, if you are liable to 'fly off the handle', as they say, then you have a problem.

Hidden conflicts within a person will frequently show up in an excessive use of alcohol, for example. You (or your friend) may claim to be just a social drinker, but look into your heart and ask yourself if you (or he) drinks just to be sociable, and for no other reason. Does he drink to deal with his own anxiety about some aspect of your relationship? What about other motives? Are you slavishly going along with everything your friend wants because you are afraid that he will reject you if you exhibit a bit of independence? Getting to know yourself and your partner is a life-long process. The process may never be complete, but some good degree of self-understanding and understanding of others is essential before you consider getting together with

97

someone on a long-term basis. Marriage won't solve your emotional problems; rather, it will tend to create two problems where before there was only one.

Particularly important, as we have been emphasizing throughout this book, is self-acceptance. If you cannot unblamingly accept yourself when you make mistakes in your relationship, you are unlikely to accept your partner when he or she does the wrong thing. You cannot really care for somebody if you hate yourself. If you blame yourself when you say or do the wrong thing, you are hardly likely to see your partner's point of view when he or she acts in a manner you consider wrong or inconsiderate. If he cannot accept himself he is likely to blame you or hate himself when things go wrong. So work on your own level of emotional instability, and choose as a partner someone who is relatively emotionally stable himself.

Communication

It may seem obvious, but the essence of a good relationship is the ability to talk to each other. If your would-be partner comes over as the strong silent type, you had better ask yourself why. He may not be the talkative kind, you think, until you see him with his pals at the leisure centre, when he talks ten to the dozen! So, if your friend is tight-lipped, especially when he is with you, find out why he appears so afraid to open his mouth when you are around. He may be a great sport and popular with his club friends, but if he seldom opens up when he is with you, who needs him? Living under the same roof day after day might not be the ideal scene for scintillating conversation, but you can realistically expect *some* degree of mutual sharing of feelings and ideas at least *some* of the time!

What if you discover that, in spite of all your efforts to create a close and loving relationship, it is obvious that the two of you have too many basic incompatibilities? Our advice is that you should consider any other kind of relationship that you or your friend can devise, except the one where you actually live together. For the chances are that you and he are just not going to make it.

These, then, are some of the more important things to bear in mind when you are interested in finding a suitable partner for a good marriage or long-term relationship. You can, no doubt, add several other desirable criteria – obvious ones such as good health, adequate earning power, as well as attributes you personally find important, such as companionship, sex-drive, ambition, and so on. With a clear idea of what you are looking for in a potential partner, the next question is how you go about finding such a person. The following suggestions are mainly intended for women, but men are by no means excluded.

How to look for a partner: the pick-up

If you wanted to buy a new dress for some important occasion, a wedding, for example, you would normally spend a good deal of time in choosing your outfit. You would visit several stores or boutiques and try on numerous garments until you were satisfied you had got exactly what you were looking for. Similarly, if you thought of doing a course in art, you would do some background reading or research and brief yourself on what was available in your area by way of art colleges or teaching facilities, and talk to your friends to see what advice they could supply you with before you finally enrolled yourself. No one would think it at all odd if you took the initiative in these matters. Yet, when it comes to looking for a suitable mate or partner with a view to marriage or creating some other good living-together arrangement, which is one of the most important 'courses' you could undertake, the generally accepted rules you are expected to follow are very different! We make no apology for the fact that the views and advice you will find in this book are somewhat unconventional, to say the least. But they do work well, as numerous people can confirm who have actually carried out our recommendations.

'What's wrong with the usual methods of meeting the kind of partner I'm looking for?' you might well ask. 'Nothing much', we would reply, 'except that dances, cocktail parties, evening classes, church groups and so on are so very inefficient!' By all means use these methods if you will, but your chances of meeting at those events the kind of person you would really like to meet are pretty slim. Why so? Well, the person you are looking for is special, special to you. By the same token, your special partner, when you find him, will also have his own idea of what attributes he is looking for in his 'ideal' mate; and they may not necessarily be the attributes you yourself possess! In other words, both you and he are highly selective. It follows that you are going to have to audition quite a few men before you can expect, on the law of averages, to meet just one who will meet your requirements, and you his. And it follows from that that you would be wise to adopt the fastest and most efficient way there is to maximize your chances of meeting the kind of person you want, with the minimum waste of time. And that way is the *pick-up*!

In this method, you approach a likely looking prospect and spontaneously pick him up right where you see him: in the street, on a bus, in a train, in a park, in a restaurant, anywhere he happens to be. One caution though: don't take undue risks and expose yourself to danger. So what are the advantages of meeting men this way?

First, it's the fastest technique there is. Going to dances, parties and so on takes time. You have to get dressed and go out to where the event is taking place. Not so with the spontaneous pick-up! You are already in position, as it were, and likely to see lots of men around, unless, of course, you happen to be visiting your sister in a convent. So, you approach the person and start up a conversation on some pretext or other. It's not time-consuming, and you've got instant companionship.

Second, you are employing the most selective technique known. At parties and discos you don't have a random sample of men to choose from. You tend to find a self-selected crowd at these functions, and even more so at lectures and church meetings. But in the street, or wherever you decide to do your man-seeking, you have a very large randomly mixed sample of men to choose from. Consequently, if you persist in looking, your chances of finding the calibre of man you are looking for are greater than in any other method of meeting people.

Third, by taking the initiative yourself, you avoid the disadvantages of the passive type of pick-up. If you just walk or sit around waiting for some man to pick you up, you run the risk of being taken up by some undesirable types who are interested in only one thing. He may be a rapist, or a murderer or some other kind of unpleasant character who is not out for your own good. If, however, you do the picking up, and actively *select* and make the first overtures to some attractive-looking man, he is much less likely to be the peculiar or dangerous type. And if you do this within the view of others then you reduce the risk of danger even more. If you discover after a few minutes conversation that you have made a mistake, you can always plead another appointment or something like that, and leave him. When you do eventually find an interesting prospect, as you will if you persist in looking and looking, you can then go to a café, for example, and talk. Select a setting where other people are around for extra safety. Find out as much as you can about him, his type of work, where he lives, his tastes in food, music or whatever. You are not there to pass the time of day with him. Your object should be to acquire as much information about your prospect as you can, while giving him at the same time a fair amount of information about yourself. Then, depending on how well things are going, you can exchange phone numbers and arrange to meet again in some public place later so that you can continue the getting-to-know-you process.

'Oh, I couldn't do that!' we can imagine some of you saying. 'What would people think of me if I went up to strange men and started to make friendly overtures to them?' Well, maybe your maiden aunt would take a dim view of your behaviour, and some of your friends would think you 'pushy' and brazen. But why inhibit yourself by what others think of you? Their thoughts, or even their disapproving words, aren't going to hurt you. Some of your friends will even secretly admire you and wish they had the 'guts' to do the same thing themselves. 'But what about the men? What will they think about a woman who makes overtures to them?' you may ask. We can tell you: most of them will be surprised and delighted! Many men who have been rejected themselves and are now loath to risk being rejected again, will be particularly glad to see you taking the risks which they theoretically should be taking themselves. They will admire your spirit and be only too pleased to be picked up! 'Won't a few men think me a bit of a hussy, or even a tart for approaching them directly?' you may ask. Probably, yes! But then, who needs them? The more you go ahead and take the initiative, the more you help to weaken that anti-feminist, male-supremacist attitude that has been responsible for putting women down in the past, and which unfortunately is still prevalent.

Finally, by going ahead and actively seeking out the kind of partner you really want to meet, using the spontaneous pick-up technique, you not only give yourself a head start over your more inhibited competition, but you give yourself the best possible chance of finding the kind of person who will really turn you on, and with the minimum waste of time. Remember, in the dating and mating game, time is important. The greater the number of potential prospects you can audition in the time available to you, the better are your chances of netting yourself the most suitable partner for you. Good luck!

SUMMARY POINTS FOR CHAPTER 6

(1) In Western culture, and probably in others, too, several popular myths prevail about love. These often reflect the kinds of common, deep-seated irrational beliefs which are the cause of emotional problems. Love itself, or rejection, is not the cause of the problem.

(2) With regard to rejection, these irrational beliefs may be briefly summarised thus:

    (a) 'I *should not* have been rejected by you and the fact that you have rejected me proves that there is something radically wrong with me and I will probably never find somebody like you again.'

    (b) 'Conditions should be arranged so that I'm always able to win the love of anyone I want without too much trouble. When conditions are against me, life becomes awful, and I can't stand it because I'll always be miserable!'

(3) These irrational notions can be shown not only to be untenable but positively unhelpful in enabling a person rejected in love to

101

get over the rejection and find another more suitable partner.

(4) Unconditional self-acceptance is an important prerequisite for success in love; you are not a worthless or inadequate person if you fail to win the love you want.

(5) Adults don't *need* love.

(6) There are two types of jealousy: rational and irrational. The latter is brought on by the various irrational demands you make upon yourself and your partner. For example, how can anyone *guarantee* to love you indefinitely? And how realistic is it to *demand* eternal devotion from someone you care for? By learning to think rationally, you can save yourself much needless emotional turmoil.

(7) Among the qualities you should preferably look for in a partner are compatibility, emotional stability, and the ability to communicate.

(8) If you want to maximise your chances of finding a suitable partner, it is important that you take the initiative and select from a large sample. Use every opportunity to meet potentially suitable partners. Try the 'pick-up' method, but don't take any undue risks.

7

Shame and Embarrassment

The Master of Ceremonies has just introduced you, the guest speaker, to the assembled audience, already eagerly awaiting your advertised lecture. The waiters have cleared the tables, and as you rise to your feet, a sea of upturned faces gazes expectantly towards you. 'Ladies and Gentlemen', you begin, as the applause dies away. Then . . . *silence*! Not a word passes your lips as you desperately strive to remember what it was you intended to say. Several seconds tick away as you stand there, silent and helpless as your mind frantically searches for those opening remarks you had previously rehearsed so well but nothing comes out. And then the stunning realization hits you. Your mind has gone completely blank! You can't even remember your name! You feel the blood rushing to your face, your breathing becomes difficult and your throat constricts as you glance to the right, then to the left, feeling like a trapped animal. But there is no escape! You just stand there, conscious of a slight titter of amusement, a restless shuffle of feet coming from somewhere among the audience, and wishing the floor would open and swallow you up. The emotion you feel is one of intense embarrassment. Have you ever experienced that situation, or something like it?

Or consider this. Imagine you have prepared a dinner party for a small group of friends. You have gone to the trouble of cooking a large joint of roast beef. As you carve the beef and serve your guests, you become aware that the buzz of conversation has ceased and an unaccountable silence has descended upon the room. You look up, and as you glance round the table, one of the guests whom you know well catches your eye: 'Have you forgotten?' she asks, looking at you pointedly. 'We're all strict vegetarians!' The emotion you experience in this situation is intense shame.

As in the previous vignette, you feel very uncomfortable. Perhaps you blush to the roots of your hair, or your mouth goes dry. You just wish that the floor would open up and remove you from the scene. Some people, faced with this, or a similar situation, might well rush out of the dining room and proceed to have a fit of hysterics in the kitchen!

Why do you think that, faced with these situations, most people would feel acutely embarrassed in the first one and very ashamed in the second? If you asked your friends that question, you would probably be told: 'Well, wouldn't *anybody* feel embarrassed if they got up to make a speech and couldn't remember anything they intended to say? And as for serving up a roast beef dinner to a group of confirmed vegetarians at a dinner party – well, what a social gaffe that was! How could you *not* feel ashamed of yourself for making such a ridiculous mistake! It wasn't that the guests were strangers, they were your friends whose tastes you knew well; and yet you go and forget such an important matter as their being vegetarian!'

If you asked us why most people faced with these situations would feel acutely embarrassed in the first case and very ashamed in the second, our answer would be: 'It isn't the situation which creates your embarrassment, or shame, but the irrational beliefs you hold about revealing an inept piece of behaviour in public. In a moment we will show you what these irrational beliefs are. Meanwhile, we would observe that because we are fallible, error-prone human beings, we can hardly avoid acting stupidly or ineptly from time to time and incurring the scorn of others for having displayed our weakness publicly. But what we claim can be avoided are the uncomfortable – and quite unnecessary – feelings of shame and embarrassment which often accompany publicly perceived incidents of socially incompetent behaviour.' To support our claim, and possibly reduce somewhat your amazed disbelief in our assertion, let us turn our attention now to an A-B-C analysis of shame and embarrassment. We will consider embarrassment first, then go on to look at shame.

The A-B-C of shame and embarrassment

Consider the example we've just given you of embarrassment. Imagine you have risen to your feet and then your mind goes completely blank. You can't remember a single word of your speech and you just stand there desperately trying to remember something of what you had intended to say. This is point A. First of all, you make certain inferences about your predicament:

(1) 'I am acting stupidly in front of all these people who have come to hear me address them.'
(2) 'The audience have spotted that I have forgotten what I was going to talk to them about.'
(3) 'They're probably thinking: "What a dumbo this person is! Did you ever see anybody looking so stupid!" '

Now, at point C, you feel very ashamed as you stand there. Why? Because you *agree* with your audience's presumed negative evaluation of you! This is point B. You are telling yourself: 'They can see I'm no good and they're right. I am a complete idiot.'

'But doesn't the conclusion that I am a complete idiot follow logically from those three inferences?' you may ask. Answer: 'No, not necessarily. Why do you *have* to agree with the audience's negative evaluation of you as a person? You see, you not only think that they are taking a dim view of your behaviour (which they are entitled to do), but you also think that they are also condemning *you* for acting so ineptly. Do you have to accept their condemnation of you, as a person, if indeed they are condemning you in this way?' Think about it. Almost anybody would agree that your inability to give your speech on cue was unfortunate. Some would also consider that you had revealed a personal weakness, although not everyone would. You could easily blackout for more than one reason. Extreme anxiety could produce a momentary blackout, for example. Some of your audience might know that and feel sorry for you, rather than critical of you. But let's suppose that your audience, almost to a man, thought you were some kind of nincompoop. Unless you agreed with them, what could possibly create that feeling of intense embarrassment? Remember, external events – things that happen outside your head – may contribute to, but cannot cause you to feel, embarrassment, or anything else for that matter. You create your own feelings by the way you evaluate or think about what is happening to you.

Thus, what would you have to believe about the situation we have just described in order for you to feel intensely embarrassed about it? The answer is something like: 'I must not reveal any weakness in public. I must do well, and be liked, especially by my audience here. I must not reveal how anxious I am to go down well with my audience. And when I fail to come up to my own, and what I consider to be their demands, then I am no good.' It is this self-denigration which is the essence of embarrassment.

'That's all very well', you might say, 'but if I act stupidly in public, like falling flat on my face when I'm trying to create a good impression, am I not entitled to curse myself for being so idiotic? You don't expect me to pat myself on the back and think, "What a jolly good fellow I am, I really screwed that one up!" Or should I say, "Oh, what the hell, what does it matter if I make an utter mess of my speech?" '

Once again, our answer is: 'No. You are certainly entitled to curse yourself for acting ineptly, but why bother? Aren't you already feeling sufficiently unhappy about your performance without giving yourself an extra dose of misery with your self-castigation? What good will that do you? Your failure to deliver your speech is one big pain in the neck; but why give yourself a second pain in the gut by telling yourself what a stinker you are? And as for pretending it doesn't matter, you know you are only lying to yourself, because you know well enough that it *does* matter; you wouldn't be so anxious to do a good job there if you really thought it was not all that important.'

'Well, what could I say to myself, so as not to feel embarrassed then, when I become over-anxious and make an ass of myself?' you might retort. First, note that you do not make an ass of *yourself*: you only act asininely. When you denigrate yourself, you are equating yourself with your actions. We have been at pains to point out several times in this book that you are not the same thing as your behaviour. Your essence or 'self' is not something that can be rated or measured in any way. You are a process, a constantly changing, living process with a great many aspects, qualities, traits and behaviours. Some of these changing characteristics may be evaluated as good or bad in terms of some external goal or standard, but your total being is unmeasurable and cannot be equated with any particular action, good or bad, that you may perform in your lifetime.

To answer (and rephrase) your question, 'What could I say to myself so as not to feel embarrassed when I behave asininely?' we would suggest that you examine and change your irrational beliefs (at point B) about the situation, and the inferences you made about the situation as follows.

'I don't like the fact that I've failed to make the speech I was billed to make. The audience are disappointed with my performance, and so am I. Nor do I like the possibility that many of those in my audience may think badly of me for acting so ineptly. But there is no reason why I must not have behaved in that unfortunate manner and there is no reason why those people in the audience must not think badly of me. That is their prerogative, but I don't have to agree with them and think badly of *me*. It's a pity I failed, and it is probably because I haven't yet overcome my anxiety that I failed on the occasion. But it isn't terrible, and I choose to accept myself as a fallible human being for acting in this way.'

If you changed your irrational self-condemning beliefs to these more rational beliefs, your feeling would be one of regret, not embarrassment. Also, without the incapacitating effects of intense embarrassment (blushing, sweating, etc.), you would be able to recover sufficiently to make some kind of response, perhaps a joking remark, to get the audience on your side, until you relaxed enough to find your memory had returned and you could get on with your address. Or, if that strategy was not practicable, you could calmly apologize for inconveniencing those present, perhaps offering a word or two of explanation for the unfortunate situation in which you found yourself. In addition, your refusal to upset yourself would encourage you to participate further in similar social events.

By contrast, embarrassing yourself tends to result in your removing yourself from the 'social spotlight'. You think to yourself: 'I'll never be able to face these people again. They'll remember me for a long time and talk about me as "that idiot who came to give us a talk and couldn't remember a word of what he had to say". I just could not bear to stand in front of them again.' In other words, embarrassment will act as a brake on your involvement in social events which remind you of your previous experience, whereas a feeling of regret will encourage you to attend such events and even accept further invitations to speak. When you experience regret, you don't put yourself on the line; you feel sorry for your inept or inappropriate behaviour, but you do not put yourself down for having behaved poorly. That is the crucial difference between regret and embarrassment. Now, let's turn our attention to shame.

Shame – and how to attack it

Shame and embarrassment occur when you find yourself agreeing with the negative evaluations that you think others place upon you when you act weakly or stupidly in public. The same type of inferences you made when you embarrassed yourself are present when you feel ashamed. The difference is that in shame, the personal weakness you reveal in public is regarded as more serious than one over which you might become embarrassed. Incidentally, some people confuse shame with guilt, and even the dictionary equates shame with guilt and mortification. This is probably because shame and guilt produce the same kind of physical effects; they both spring from the same kind of ideas, the core idea being the self-denigration which is at the root of a great deal of emotional disturbance. The difference between shame and guilt is that shame comes from receiving others' disapproval, while guilt comes from receiving one's own disapproval. Both shame and guilt are extremely unhelpful to you! We have already shown you how to overcome feelings of guilt. We now propose to show you how to free yourself from shame. In RET, we take the view that you can stubbornly refuse to feel ashamed of anything. Anything? Yes, *anything*.

Let's take the example we gave you of a dinner party which goes wrong. Imagine you have invited a few friends round to dinner. You prepare them a lovely roast beef dinner, completely forgetting that your friends are strict vegetarians. When one of them reminds you of this fact, you feel ashamed and hardly know what to do with yourself. How did you get from feeling calm and confident one minute to feeling ashamed the next?

Your inferences (at point A) are much the same as before. You begin with:

(1) 'I have acted stupidly in front of my friends.'
(2) 'They have observed at first hand my error in serving them with a

107

meal they could not eat. (If you had prepared and served the meal in your kitchen where you would not have been observed, and had suddenly recalled that your friends were vegetarians, you could have scratched the whole menu and started afresh to prepare a meal more suited to your guests' tastes and offered a plausible excuse for the delay. In that case you would not have felt ashamed, merely annoyed and irritated over your forgetfulness.)

(3) 'They are thinking "How could he be so stupid as to serve us a roast beef meal! Surely he knows we are vegetarian. What an idiot he is!" '

Your acute feeling of shame, however, does not stem from the situation at point A. As in every kind of emotional upset, your upset feelings at point C stem from the irrational beliefs you hold about what has happened at point A, and the inferences you made about this event. The following are typical of your beliefs at point B:

(1) 'I must succeed and be seen as competent and be approved of by every significant person in my life.'
(2) 'If I fail to act competently and adequately and thereby incur the disapproval of others who have witnessed my inadequacy, that proves I'm a pretty hopeless individual.'
(3) 'Once people see that I'm no good, they will remember it, and I'll never be able to face them again.'

How to surrender your shame-creating beliefs

How do you get rid of the shame? You could do as some people do, and immerse yourself in some kind of diversionary activity. We don't recommend it, but you could throw yourself into making yourself extremely busy in some way. Diverting yourself from feelings of shame is a low-level palliative solution and, because it does not get to the root of your attitude of shame, it will do nothing in the longer term to help you get rid of your shame-creating propensities. We advise that you undertake something much harder, but ultimately more rewarding than diverting yourself. You will see what we have in mind for you in a minute.

But first, see if you can challenge and dispute those irrational ideas which create and sustain your shameful feelings. Such powerful feelings don't just materialize out of nothing, you know. Like anxiety, guilt, anger and depression, you create your feelings of shame from the set of basic ideas or philosophies which you bring to each situation you encounter as you go through life. You could dispute the three irrational shame-creating ideas given at the end of the previous section as follows.

'It is fine to succeed and achieve competence and mastery in my chosen field, because material and other kinds of rewards may follow. But where is it written that I absolutely *must* succeed in whatever I do, and win the approval of significant people in my life? There is no evidence that I *must* do this. "Must" implies a law of the universe, and if such a law existed I could hardly avoid succeeding in everything I tackled, and I would be practically guaranteed to win the approval of every person significant to me. Clearly no such law exists. However, it would be preferable for me to succeed and be approved of; preferable, but not essential.

'If I fail to act adequately, and as a result of my inadequacy other people look down on me, why does that make me a hopeless or worthless individual? Am I the same thing as my acts? Even if I frequently screw up on important tasks, how does that make me a total failure? How can the past ever prove anything about the future? Neither my failure to act adequately, nor the disapproval of others, says anything about me as a person. I am a human being who sometimes does well and sometimes does badly. These statements are factual and can be verified. Moreover, my past behaviour is no guarantee of my future behaviour. If that were the case, I would be obliged to go on repeating the same patterns of behaviour, like an automaton, for the rest of my life. Once again, it is a verifiable fact that one's future is not merely a repetition of one's past. I cannot, therefore, be a total failure just because I screw up once in a while on important tasks. People can and do change. I cannot, therefore, legitimately be assessed as a hopeless or worthless individual on the basis of my poor acts; for my acts are merely aspects of me, not the whole of me. Given this, I can accept myself as a fallible human being who has acted inadequately on this occasion.

'Some people might rate me negatively on account of my poor or incompetent behaviour, but why should I link my self-assessment with theirs? I can objectively assess my behaviour and try to correct my deficiencies by training, or by working to reduce or eliminate my self-defeating traits. But at the end of the day, I am *me*; a fallible, error-prone individual who will frequently act poorly or inadequately; but I need never down myself, my being, for acting badly, even if others do put me down and rate me negatively.'

If you persist with these challenges to your shame-creating beliefs you will help yourself acquire a more self-accepting philosophy. However, please do not expect quick results! Your propensity to feel ashamed or embarrassed won't melt away overnight, even if you regularly challenge and dispute the irrational ideas which create and sustain them. In discussing anxiety (Chapter 2) you may recall that we encouraged you to force yourself into doing what you were irrationally afraid to do, at the same time as you worked on changing your anxiety-creating ideas. By encouraging you to take risks and succeed in achieving what you had previously considered too anxiety-provoking, you were able to overcome your extreme anxiety and replace it with rational concern. Confidence comes with doing. Getting started is often the hardest part in any difficult but worthwhile activity. Now, since we attach great importance in RET to encouraging you to *act* against your self-defeating attitudes and behaviours, as well as helping you to think through your irrational ideas and replace them with more sensible views, we are going to describe a few exercises you can carry out practically anywhere. We call these exercises 'shame-attacking exercises' for reasons which will become obvious. For that is exactly what they are. They are designed to get you moving and acting against your ingrained shame- and embarrassment-creating attitudes, which have held you back for so long from doing many things you would have liked to do but refrained from doing because you considered them too embarrassing or shameful.

Some shame-attacking exercises

We suggest that you take someone along with you on some of these exercises if you think there is a possibility that you will get 'cold feet' and opt out of doing them at the last minute. But if you can do them on your own, so much the better. The function of your companion is solely to make sure you do the exercises, not to give you 'moral support' or encouragement. If you do opt out and fail to do an exercise, you can arrange with your companion to penalize you in some way. Ask him to hold on to a large sum of money for you and give it back only if you complete the exercise – if you don't he is to donate it to some political or religious cause you detest. If you find an assignment too easy, go on to try something more difficult. We do not believe, in RET, in making things easy for you because that only reinforces your philosophy of low frustration tolerance, your belief that life mustn't be too difficult! A word of caution before you begin: do not do anything dangerous or against the law. We don't want you to lose your job or get yourself arrested or end up in gaol! Also, don't do anything that will unduly alarm other people, even though the purpose is to encourage them to think of you as stupid or outrageous.

There are two purposes to these exercises. First, doing them gives you an experience of learning that nothing terrible will happen to you if people laugh at you or point at you and shake their heads. Second, doing them gives you the opportunity of accepting yourself as a fallible human being in the face of others' criticism of you.

Exercise No. 1

Go up to someone in a public place where there are plenty of people around and say to that person: 'Excuse me, I've just come out of the loony bin, could you tell me which day it is today?' If you get a response (and you keep on trying until you do!), you thank the person and say: 'I want to sing you a song, I used to be a great opera star, you know.'

If the person you speak to laughs at you, or calls you a rude name, that is his or her prerogative, but you don't have to go along with their negative evaluation. If you feel ashamed or humiliated, look for the irrational beliefs which make you feel that way. Then challenge and dispute them until you see that it is not your action or the other person's response to it that upsets you but the way you think about it. If you practise this a few times you will reach a point where you can tolerate a derogatory response without unduly upsetting yourself about it.

Exercise No. 2

Go up to some attractive-looking member of the opposite sex and ask him or her for a date. Don't do this in a place where you are likely to be accepted! Don't try it in a bar, for example. The whole idea is to ask for a date in circumstances where you are almost certain to be rejected, because then you can see that nothing horrible happens to you when you are rejected. No matter how often you get rejected, you are never a rejectee! Do this exercise several times until you really see that there's nothing humiliating about being turned down. Nobody can humiliate you – unless you let them.

Your humiliation comes from belittling yourself. When you are rejected, it usually means that the other person is not interested in you for a number of reasons, some of which may have nothing to do with you. Everyone, including you, has a right to his or her preferences, and you need not assume that their likes say anything about you as a person. So practise accepting yourself in the face of the unwanted and undesirable rejection.

Exercise No. 3

Go for a ride by public transport, and, making sure there are at least some other passengers in the vehicle, call out the stops, in a loud voice! If you can, use the London underground, and call out the stations so that everyone can hear you: 'Regent's Park! Regent's Park! The home of London Zoo! See the big elephants!'

If you see passengers giggling and looking at you as if you were crazy, think: 'I am acting foolishly, but that does not make me a foolish person. Therefore, when I unintentionally screw up in real life and people think badly of me, I can accept that I failed to act well on this occasion but I am not a foolish or worthless person for having acted badly or unwisely.'

Exercise No. 4

Go into a supermarket wearing some outlandish clothes. These days, what is considered outlandish in one area may be almost *de rigeur* in another. So use your judgement. If you are a male, obtain a woman's wig, stick a big colourful bow in it and put it on your head. Then spend at least ten minutes walking about in the store at a time when there are a lot of shoppers around. If people laugh at you, let them! Convince yourself that even if you *look* silly, that doesn't mean that you *are* silly. Show yourself that whatever others may think of your behaviour, you don't have to belittle yourself, although you can agree that your *behaviour* may be laughter-provoking.

You may overhear one or two people muttering about some people having abysmal taste in clothes, or having low standards in public decorum. There are, of course, standards of dress and behaviour in public, and it is rational to observe these standards. However, there may be times when you turn up for a function of some sort 'improperly dressed'. Taste and fashion in clothes is largely a matter of definition. If you present yourself at a gathering dressed in such a way as to receive adverse comment from others present, you can accept that you erred in your choice of 'gear', but that is all it is: an error of judgement which in no way makes you a socially incompetent person. Stares of disapproval are disadvantageous, but they'll hardly kill you.

Exercise No. 5

Here's one for the men. Go into a shop where they sell condoms. One of the large multiple chemist shops will do. Arrive at the counter where the condoms are displayed when the store is really busy. Try to attract the attention of one of the counter assistants, preferably a female. Then, pointing to the condoms, ask in a voice loud enough to be heard by everyone else in the vicinity: 'Are these condoms here the only type you have? Haven't you got the ribbed and dotted ones – you know, the kind that give the woman extra excitement?'

And for the women, go into a shop where they sell all manner of sex aids. Wait until there are at least one or two other people around within earshot, then go up to an assistant and demand in a loud voice: 'I want a double-ended vibrator with independent multi-speed control, and it must be at least 10 inches long!'

Maybe some people will view your behaviour as outrageous, but you won't be hanged for it. So you acted in a way which might be interpreted by some people as outrageous or at least in poor taste. On the other hand, some other people might secretly admire you! In real life, your opinions may well 'outrage' some people. Some people might take exception to some of the things written in this book. If you hide your true opinions for fear of disapproval, rather than on account of some actual penalty you may incur, you are clinging to the irrational idea that your opinions and tastes must always be acceptable to others, and it's awful if they are not because that would make you worthless. Can you rationally support that idea? Of course you can't, and this exercise and the previous one will help to get the point home to you in a manner you are unlikely to forget.

These are just a few suggestions for ways of attacking your tendency to become embarrassed, or ashamed, or shy, or humiliated when you do things which other people consider shameful or ludicrous, or stupid. Even when you do rate your own actions as stupid, unwise or inadequate, as you will probably do from time to time, you can learn never to belittle or denigrate yourself for your poor behaviour. And if you give up denigrating yourself when you behave poorly, you will find it much easier to give up condemning other people when they do stupid or annoying acts, whether intentional or not. Learn to accept yourself as a fallible human being who will never become perfect, but who has a right to life and happiness. By all means work at changing your less desirable habits, using the techniques we have taught you in this book, and acquire a more realistic, self-helping attitude to life. Risk-taking is a part of life, and you chance defeat as well as success. But if you never take any risks for fear of failure or fear of disapproval, you will tend to lead a fairly inhibited, low-level kind of existence, and may never discover what you would really like to do with your life. Life is not a bed of roses; it is filled with innumerable hassles. But it is not awful, or terrible. If you are sensible in taking risks, and actively seek happiness, you can accept the challenge of this difficult existence, and make it less difficult for you personally, and even exciting and enjoyable for yourself and your loved ones. What more can one ask of life?

SUMMARY POINTS FOR CHAPTER 7

(1) Whenever you act foolishly or ineptly in public and you feel embarrassed or ashamed for having publicly revealed some weakness, you may think that your embarrassment is caused by other people's expressed disapproval of your behaviour. Perhaps they deride you or dismiss you as an insensitive clot. Or they may strongly indicate that you just are not up to the level of competence you think you are.

(2) By now, we hope that your study of this book will have convinced you that, in terms of the A-B-C model of emotional disturbance, A does not and cannot cause C. A, you'll recall, stands for an activating event (such as doing something foolish in public and incurring public scorn or criticism). And C stands for your emotional reaction or, simply, the way you feel and behave immediately after your foolish act. As you now know, your emotional consequences at C are caused by B, your set of beliefs about what has happened to you at point A.

(3) In terms of our A-B-C analysis of shame and embarrassment, your feelings of shame and embarrassment stem from your *agreement* with your audience's presumed negative evaluation of you. In effect, you are telling yourself: 'They can see I'm no good and they're right!'

(4) Can you rationally support the proposition that because you may have acted stupidly or inappropriately in some way you are therefore a stupid person? We have aleady shown you that when you denigrate yourself you are equating your *self* with your actions and that this is irrational. Your total being is unmeasurable and cannot legitimately be equated with any particular action, good or bad.

(5) Also, your self-denigration stems from the irrational belief that says: 'I must not reveal any weakness in public. I must do well and be approved of by every person who is significant to me. And if I fail to come up to these standards I demand of myself, then I am no good.'

(6) The rational alternative to feelings of shame and embarrassment in a situation where you act incompetently is a feeling of disappointment or regret that you have failed, at least in this instance, to perform to your own or others' satisfaction. Then, without the inhibiting effects of shame or embarrassment, you can figure out how to improve your performance the next time.

(7) As a useful aid to overcoming your tendency to feel shame or embarrassment and to combat the irrational ideas which generate these negative self-evaluations, we introduced a number of activities which we urged you to carry out. We called them 'shame-attacking exercises' because that is exactly what they are designed to do: attack your feelings of shame. These exercises are useful in reinforcing your efforts to uproot the negative, self-devaluing beliefs which create and sustain feelings of shame and embarrassment, and in helping you accept yourself and work to correct your mistakes when you fail, as occasionally you will, to act as efficiently and as well as you would wish.

8
Problems of Self-Discipline

At the outset, let us make this clear: self-discipline *per se* is not a problem; it is the *lack* of it which is a disadvantage, and sometimes a serious disadvantage for anyone who chooses, as most of us do, to live and work in a modern society. Maybe if you lived on a desert island, surrounded by your eight favourite discs, and with nothing much to do all day except lie in the sun and live off the fruit of the land, a lack of self-discipline might not seem much of a hindrance. However, for most of us, reality is a very different kettle of fish. We certainly do not live in the best of all possible worlds. Difficult problems abound everywhere in this economically unstable, polluted, politically oppressive, violence-filled world teeming with billions of people all striving to stay alive and have their way as far as possible. Our world is full of hassles and we frequently have to perform disagreeable tasks just to stay alive as well as to obtain whatever real advantages from life we select to go after.

If you want to achieve a good measure of control over your own destiny, to feel that you are in the saddle, a high degree of self-discipline is practically mandatory. Not that you *have* to become self-disciplined! You don't *have* to do anything. But if you want to live a reasonably healthy life and achieve your personal goals with the minimum expenditure of time and energy, then you would be wise to make the attainment of a high degree of self-discipline one of your priorities, even, indeed, your *top* priority. Without a fair degree of self-discipline, you will tend to procrastinate and you may find yourself indulging in alcohol or other substances whenever you find life becoming 'too hard'.

In the following sections we will show you why poor self-discipline can be a serious disadvantage to you in the business of living, how it is caused, and what you can do to overcome it so that you can lead a happier, more satisfying existence. But first, let's investigate why good self-discipline takes time and work to develop. As you will see, avoiding difficult situations may bring you immediate pleasure, but in the long run it can be very expensive and even painful.

Where does self-discipline come from?

We're certainly not born with it! From the moment we leave the womb, we begin the long and difficult journey towards adulthood, the state where we reach independence from our parents and achieve the ability to function as autonomous individuals in society. As infants, we know only our bodily wants and the need for their immediate satisfaction. We would not survive if any of our vital needs were delayed for long. Consequently, most of us grow up expecting to have our desires gratified fairly rapidly. The discomforts of hunger and thirst are displaced by the pleasures of being fed and bathed and comforted. We come to expect that pain and discomfort will soon give way to pleasant feelings of ease and satisfaction.

While all this instant gratification may have been good for us as babies because it promoted our survival, it has certain hidden costs. As we grow up, we find that the world around us no longer makes the immediate satisfaction of our wants its top priority. We have to learn to wait! Later, we not only have to wait but also have to work for the satisfaction of many of our daily wants. We seldom get what we want the minute we ask for it. This transition from the immediate satisfaction of desires to the postponement of immediate gratification for the purpose of obtaining some more important satisfaction in the longer term, is one of the most difficult stages in the growth towards maturity. Some people, unfortunately, never quite make it. They remain babies all their lives, because they fail to accept that they cannot have every wish instantly fulfilled; and when their wishes are not instantly fulfilled – as most frequently they are not or cannot be – they scream and whine about how 'unfair' the world is, and how they can't *stand* being treated in such a horrible manner!

We shall presently show you the basic irrational ideas which sabotage your ability to deal adequately with the world as it is. The point we wish to make here is that our human tendency to avoid pain or discomfort by taking the route which promises instant relief is biologically-based, in the sense that it once had proven survival value for us in our dependent infancy. However, although it is sensible and often life-preserving to avoid pain and various kinds of discomfort which may mar your enjoyment of life, the rules of the game change when you leave childhood behind and begin to learn to stand on your own two feet. Instead of seeking instant gratification of your desires, you will frequently find it necessary to take a longer-term view of your situation and to put up with a certain amount of inconvenience, pain or discomfort in the present, in order to reap the advantage of achieving a more comfortable situation in the future. For example, you may disregard your doctor's advice to have a surgical operation now, because you feel anxious about going into hospital to undergo surgery. But you may well find later that, by postponing treatment to a later date, you have to undertake a more serious operation with less chance of a successful outcome, followed by a long and possibly painful period of recuperation and convalescence. You thus end up experiencing more anxiety and discomfort that you would if you had decided to go for the operation in the first place. To choose present pain for future gain isn't easy; it goes 'against the grain', as they say. But the easy way out is often just that: the way out of a happier, more enjoyable existence. In RET, we believe in helping people to survive and live as happily as they can in this one life they have on earth. And since we also believe strongly in efficiency, which means in this context living rationally, we strongly recommend anyone wishing to live rationally to acquire a good degree of self-discipline. In fact, we would go so far as to claim that unless you do acquire a high degree of self-discipline, you will find it almost impossible to live rationally and happily in this highly irrational world of ours.

Poor self-discipline – the consequences

When you think it is easier to avoid a difficult task, such as writing a really comprehensive report for your boss, than it is to face all the hard work involved in getting the report written and presented to your boss by the target date, you are the victim of poor self-discipline. You know that a well-presented report delivered on time will mean you are likely to get a good positive annual appraisal and will help further your career prospects. You know you can produce the kind of report the boss and the board are looking for. But you also know you are going to have to work extra hours to assemble all the data needed to back up the recommendations the report will put forward. You know you are going to incur some unpopularity with your staff because you will be leaning on them to get the various section inputs produced, checked, approved and typed on time. It is a lot of hassle! And you know, too, that if you didn't produce the report on time, you could make a number of excuses, like being short-staffed most of the time due to illnesses, people leaving the firm, lack of co-operation from outside sources, and so on. They're not likely to sack you if that report is not ready when the boss wants it. So you'll still get by. It won't entirely be your fault if the report isn't ready by the time the board want it. It would be nice, very nice, if you could drop the completed report on your boss's desk a few days before the board are due to meet. You know you are in line for promotion, and a good report will certainly not do your career prospects any harm. But it is so much work! 'It shouldn't be so hard!' you say to yourself. And when you see how Jones in the finance department seems to get his reports out on time each year with apparently so little effort, you tell yourself: 'It isn't fair! Why should he have such an easy time, when I have to work so very hard all the year round just to keep up with the work!' And so, you drop a few hints around that, this year, your department will be late with its annual report. Not your fault, of course! There are many extenuating circumstances; but at the end of the day, your boss explains to his board why your report is not to hand, and he makes certain entries in your personal appraisal file. One day, you notice your name is not on the list of candidates invited to appear before the promotion board. What caused you to lose out when the time came to draw up the list of candidates for promotion? An angry boss? Unhelpful colleagues? Shortage of staff?

Low Frustration Tolerance

Actually, none of these factors was the real cause of your losing out on the promotion stakes. You lost out primarily because of your Low Frustration Tolerance (LFT). LFT has an immense effect on human affairs. You have already seen in previous chapters how it sustains and makes worse various kinds of emotional disturbance. But LFT is also the primary cause of other problems such as avoidance of hard work, over-eating, and over-indulgence in alcohol and other drugs. Procrastination is one of the principal results of LFT. The consequence of procrastination is to make the attainment of your objectives much harder than would otherwise have been the case had you buckled down and carried out the necessary work in the first instance. To procrastinate is like throwing sand into the works of an otherwise well-functioning machine. You get increased wear and tear, the job generally takes longer to complete, and the machine may well seize up altogether! Procrastination, and poor self-discipline which causes and accompanies procrastination, are the twin saboteurs of your ability to lead an efficient and happy existence. There are other self-sabotaging philosophies which hinder and block your efforts to achieve your important goals in life – and we shall discuss these presently – but LFT is the prime culprit. So let's see what you can do to raise your ability to tolerate frustrating conditions and give yourself scope to deal adequately with the inevitable frustrations and hassles of everyday living.

When you recognize that to obtain some future gain, you have to undertake present pain, and you believe that pain is *too* awful to bear, and *too* much to undertake, you are experiencing LFT. Suppose we consider that report again. To begin with, you have the quite reasonable belief that: 'This report is going to mean a lot of hard work and it will be difficult to get it out on time. I wish I was not responsible for it and didn't have to do it.' These are factual statements; they can be confirmed and verified. But then, you go on to the quite irrational belief that: 'It's not only hard, it's *too* hard! I *can't stand* it – all those long grinding hours – and at the end of it, there's no guarantee that the boss will accept it, or that the board will approve it. This situation should not exist.' The consequence of this irrational thinking is desperate avoidance of getting involved with the preparation of your report. You put off making a start until you can prove there is no way the report can be produced by the required date. So you escape from the pain associated with producing the report and feel a sense of relief. But only for a time! The board will set a new date for your report, and will make a special note that you failed to carry out your assignment by the date originally set for it. You know that your failure to meet the original deadline will not do your career any good and you will begin to worry about *that*, in addition to experiencing further anxiety about getting the report out by the revised date. Escaping the pain of buckling down to the task you were originally set has only put you in a situation where you now have a double dose of pain to bear where before you had only one! You will find innumerable instances in life where procrastination makes a difficult situation worse, rather than better. Your problems won't just simply disappear because you have put off tackling them; sooner or later, you will have to face them again – along with a few new ones you failed to foresee arising as a consequence of avoiding tackling the first lot! 'How do you get over the problems of procrastination, then, seeing it has so many disadvantages?' you may well ask. By challenging the irrational, self-defeating ideas which create your procrastinating behaviour and replacing them with sensible, workable ideas which will help you develop the self-disciplined strategies you will need to carve out a more rewarding life for yourself. Since LFT is the prime culprit behind your procrastination, we will deal with LFT first, then go on to examine those other factors which frequently overlap with LFT.

Disputing your LFT beliefs

By now you may be familiar with our RET method of scientifically questioning and logically examining commonly held ideas to see if they are really true. LFT arises from the belief that life conditions must not be difficult and that it is easier to avoid facing many of life's difficulties and responsibilities than to undertake more rewarding forms of self-discipline. Or, otherwise stated: 'I cannot stand present pain for future gain.' Can this idea be upheld? Certainly, many people act as if they thought so! We have pointed out in previous chapters of this book that the idea that you can't stand what you don't like is nonsense. You can stand anything until you die of it! What you really mean, of course, is that you *won't* stand it – you refuse to stand or put up with whatever it is you detest. In other words, every time you put off doing something you know it would be better to do sooner rather than later because it's difficult, or boring, or a lot of hassle, you are telling yourself some variation of what we termed 'irrational belief no. 3'. You'll find it near the end of Chapter 1: 'Because it is preferable that I experience pleasure rather than pain, the world absolutely must arrange this and life is horrible, and I can't bear it, when the world does not.'

It would be nice if we could get the world always to arrange matters so that we were never inconvenienced, or that we never had to go through pain or discomfort to get what we want in life. But the world isn't like that, and life is patently unfair. Individuals and corporations alike continually make life more difficult for themselves by opting for easy short-term solutions to problems only to find sooner or later that the original problem still has to be resolved, and at considerably greater expense than if the matter had been tackled head on when it first became urgent.

We are not advocating that you try to live a spartan existence or postpone every chance you get for pleasurable enjoyment at the moment it is offered. Far from it! What we are saying is that if your common sense tells you that it would be wiser to delay pleasure, but you refuse to wait because you 'can't stand the frustration', or because you 'deserve a bit of fun', then you are acting on some variation of irrational belief no. 3.

A case of LFT

Exam time was coming up and Roger had spent the previous year studying hard for it. Roger was a student, not particularly gifted, but he worked hard, usually in fits and starts. The night before his exam, Roger and his friends discovered that Roger's favourite pop group was playing a one-night stand in a neighbouring town. It was 'the chance of a lifetime!' said Roger's friends. Roger had many of the group's discs, and frequently had them playing on his hi-fi equipment. Here at last was a chance to see and hear the group live! Roger felt some qualms about spending the night before the exam in a disco in another town. He knew it would be virtually an all-night affair. But he decided he could get back in time for the exam, just about.

Roger and his friends had a great time that night at the disco. But, as he sat down in the examination room next morning, Roger felt distinctly jaded. He had been up all night and had also had a lot to drink. The paper was not an easy one. Near the end of the time allowed for the exam, Roger discovered that he had misread one of the questions and had spent a good hour answering a question which had not been asked. Since he had struggled to answer less than half of the remaining questions, Roger slashed his pen through his paper in a fit of pique and sought permission to leave the examination room. Not surprisingly, Roger failed his course for that year and was compelled to repeat it the following year.

During counselling, Roger was shown how he had blown a full year's work because of his childish insistence on instant gratification at the expense of his more important goals. Roger easily saw the logic of his counsellor's arguments and was eventually persuaded to focus on his true priorities (which were to obtain his degree and enter accountancy) and to combat his irrational beliefs that life should not be too hard, and that life somehow 'owed him a bit of fun'.

Let's look at this belief that something can be 'too hard'. A thing is either possible or impossible. It may be physically or inherently impossible due to some law of nature; or it may be practically impossible, meaning that the materials, the tools, or the skills needed to carry out the work are not available. But, given that some task is possible, it can then be graded on a scale of difficulty from easy through moderately difficult to extremely difficult. Nowhere is there a mark which signifies 'too difficult', except in someone's head! If you find yourself thinking that something is 'too hard', remember you are only kidding yourself. Nothing can ever be 'too hard'.

You can also subject your other irrational notions to logical examination. Have you any real evidence that life *owes* you a 'bit of fun', or indeed anything? If life really did owe us what we desired, wouldn't we get it? Since most of the time we seem to get what we want only if we work for it (and sometimes not even then!) would we not be better advised to give up the belief that the world owes us anything at all?

LFT is not the only irrational attitude which leads to poor self-discipline and the various forms of procrastination. We turn our attention now to those other saboteurs of intelligent goal-directed behaviour: self-deprecation; hostility; and addiction.

Self-deprecation

A good deal of emotional disturbance is caused by people putting themselves down – denigrating themselves. We have already seen in previous chapters how this leads to anxiety, depression and feelings of worthlessness. Practically all of us have the desire to perform important tasks well, and to experience approval, respect or love from others we regard as significant to us. These desires are sensible because achieving them can bring us pleasure and enhance our lives. However, instead of sticking to these desires, instead of viewing them as strongly held preferences, we escalate them into absolutistic, dogmatic, dire necessities. 'I *should*, *ought* and *must* have what I really want!' takes over, and that's when our problems begin. If you lay a *demand* on yourself, if you absolutely insist on getting top marks from your tutor on your next written assignment, for example, and a guarantee of acclaim for your magnificent effort, and then fail to achieve it, you conclude: 'Since I failed to do what I *must* do, I rate as a no-good person.' With that philosophy, you will feel anxious at the thought of not doing an absolutely perfect job of writing, and that thought may impel you to avoid carrying out your assignment, or to leave it so late that you can hardly avoid submitting a scrappy paper. You then get off the hook by telling yourself that you could not possibly have done a perfect assignment due to the lack of time. Of course, you created your own hook to hang yourself on by your irrational demand that you write a perfect paper and win the acclaim and admiration of all and sundry in the first place. When you find yourself procrastinating on starting some task which is important to you, look for your absolutistic shoulds, oughts or musts. They are probably there in some form or other!

Hostility

Hostility and LFT frequently go hand in hand. The main irrational belief underlying hostility is: 'Other people *must* treat me fairly, kindly and considerately, and do what I want.' With that belief you are going to feel angry and resentful on those occasions (which may be numerous!) when you *don't* get treated kindly, fairly and considerately, as you insist you *must*. The manner in which hostility can lead you into procrastination may be best seen from the following example.

Jonathan, the 17-year-old son of two music teacher parents and a member of a music-loving family, was already showing promise as a violinist. He actually enjoyed playing his instrument when he felt like it but continually baulked at staying in at night to practise under his parents' supervision. Jonathan's parents were determined that their son should reach concert-playing status and to that end constantly persuaded and cajoled and harried Jonathan into more and more practice of his violin playing. The more his parents insisted, the more Jonathan resisted. He took to going out at nights for long periods with his friends. Eventually he got himself into trouble with the police over illicit drug taking. Jonathan's violin career soon fell by the wayside.

Jonathan's rebellion was a way of getting back at his parents for what he saw as an attempt to control his life. He wanted to show that *he* was in control, not his parents. Jonathan certainly had the talent to succeed as a violinist, as his parents rightly perceived, and he might well have made a name for himself one day had he practised long and hard on the instrument. As it turned out, Jonathan gave up the violin completely. It was his way of saying: 'I'll show them who's boss around here!' Jonathan's irrational belief about his parents' nagging was: 'You must treat me with more consideration and stop nagging me, and if you don't I'll spite you by giving up the violin, even if I cut off my nose in the process!'

A more rational alternative for Jonathan would have been to take the view: 'There go my parents again with their continual nagging. They're a real pain in the neck. Of course, I know it's important and in my own eventual interest to practise playing my violin daily. But if I do, it is because I want to, and not just because they insist on it. So, I'll ignore them and maybe they'll get off my back when they see that I'm doing OK and passing my music exams. But if they still bug me, tough! I can still work hard at my playing because it is in my best long-term interest to do so. I'll never like my parents' attitude, but I'm strong enough to lump it.'

You will probably spot some degree of LFT in Jonathan's attitude towards his parents. As we noted above, LFT often accompanies other unhelpful emotions like hostility. In fact, we find that most procrastination has more to do with LFT and feelings of inadequacy than spite or revenge arising from hostility. But it does happen that anger at someone's 'unfairness' occasionally causes people to procrastinate, so it is wise to be aware of it.

Addictions

Addictions take many forms. You can become addicted to drugs, to people, to playing a certain role in life, to virtually anything. Many books have been written on the subject of addiction. For our purposes we shall focus on the psychological aspects of addiction. In the popular mind, addiction is seen as some kind of chemical bond which, once established through frequent use, chains the victim to the substance believed to 'cause' the addiction for the remainder of that person's life. There is some doubt as to whether addictions really are created and maintained by some biochemical bond. What seem to be much more firmly established are the psychological mechanisms underlying every form of addiction so far known. It is to these basic psychological factors that we now direct your attention.

The psychological causes of addiction

You may usefully think of addiction, such as addiction to alcohol, in much the same way as you think of procrastination. There are striking similarities between them. Addiction is like a kind of permanent procrastination. Whereas the average procrastinator usually gets round to doing whatever has to be done sooner or later (usually later!), the person addicted to alcohol or drugs may stay addicted for months, years, even a lifetime. Stanton Peele and Archie Brodsky maintain that addiction is basically the same thing as dependency. (*Love and Addiction*, Abacus 1977) When we look into this matter of dependency we find that several irrational ideas are present – ideas with which you may now be familiar:

(1) 'I must be spared the hassles of life and it is easier to avoid than to face certain life difficulties and responsibilities.'

(2) 'When life is difficult others must help to make life less difficult for me. I need them to rely upon.'

Add to these the basic irrational ideas underlying LFT and you have a trio of powerful ideas which will strongly motivate and help create and maintain almost any form of addiction:

(3) 'Because it is preferable that I experience pleasure rather than pain, the world absolutely must arrange this and life is horrible, and I can't bear it when the world does not.'

There is a certain aptness of phrase which some drug abusers use to express their attitude towards life. 'Turn on', 'tune in', and 'drop out' are all quite accurate descriptions of what these individuals are doing; in effect they are escaping, blotting out aspects of the world which they feel they can no longer tolerate. When life seems too tough, many people who would not consider themselves addicts, turn towards artificial stimulants to disrupt boredom or help them relax after a stressful day at the office. In many ways our culture fosters dependency on drugs and stimulants and makes it easy for us to acquire them.

Taking drugs appeals to those who tend to procrastinate. Finding it difficult to acquire the skills to live a constructive, decisive kind of life, and being accustomed to dilly-dallying over all sorts of problems where any hassle is involved in overcoming them, procrastinators find it easy (in the short term) to resort to drugs to obtain the kicks they need to make life more bearable. Drug abuse is thus a defence against facing and dealing with life's problems and is self-defeating in the long-term.

Ironically, procrastinators with a pronounced feeling of self-denigration become so painfully aware and ashamed of their procrastination, that they turn to drugs to anaesthetize their self-denigration.

In effect, these unfortunate people create a secondary problem: 'I must not procrastinate and I'm no good for procrastinating' is the basic irrational belief. The consequence is that overcoming the 'original' problem of procrastination becomes twice as difficult for them.

How to change your addictive thinking

We have introduced you in previous chapters to some of the various techniques used in RET to overcome self-defeating upsetting emotions and behaviour. If you have a problem of addiction, you would be wise to employ several different methods in conjunction to help you change your thinking, feeling and behaviour away from dependency on external crutches like alcohol or drugs and towards autonomous living. Thus, you could identify and dispute the validity of the main irrational ideas set out above which lead you into dependency or addiction in the first place. For example: Look out for your musts, your demands. *Must* you be dependent on some external person or thing for a sense of personal adequacy or security? Since you cannot be sure that your external source of support and comfort will always be available when you want it, you will tend to feel even less confident of your ability to cope with your life. By learning to stand on your own feet you will learn better ways of coping. So it's hard, and you'll make mistakes. But it is not *too* hard. You can learn from your mistakes, and you can make a particular note that your failures have nothing to do with your intrinsic worth as a human being. Only you can know what you really want out of life and only you can face and solve your own living problems. Drugs don't solve anything. If you let them take over, they will only sabotage your chances of a reasonably sane and happy life.

Whenever you take a step backwards in your efforts to rid yourself of your dependence on drugs, refuse to view yourself as a worthless person or a hopeless case. It's not good that you fell back, but how does your foolish act make you a totally no-good person? Not at all! When you make a mistake, by going back to your drinking or drugs, that only proves you are fallible. But you are still an acceptable human being. Change is difficult sometimes, but in the long run it may be harder not to change.

In addition to changing your thinking about your addiction, we encourage acting against your addicting habits. You can use self-management techniques to stop drinking, for example. You can use shame-attacking exercises to help you undercut the feelings of shame, embarrassment and humiliation which are the core of so much emotional disturbance and which frequently 'drive' people to drink or drugs as a way of allaying such feelings. Details of these methods have been set out in previous chapters and you will find it useful to study

125

them again and use them in a constructive manner to help you kick your addictions and live your life in a more confident manner.

How to stop procrastinating and get started

If you have a report to prepare for your boss by a certain date, or a course essay to write and submit to your tutor before a cut-off date, and you find it difficult to make a start, apply some of the self-management techniques we described for you in earlier chapters. Once you have got going and completed a reasonable amount of the work, reward yourself in some way. But only *after*, not before, you have done the requisite amount of work! As you get down to it, think these rational thoughts to help keep you at it: 'It sure is hard work, but then there is no reason why it shouldn't be hard. If I keep my nose to the grindstone I stand a good chance of making out well with my boss or tutor. My object is to succeed this year, otherwise I'll have it all to do again next year. Where's the sense in that? Besides, the work itself isn't entirely boring; I can learn some useful things from this exercise which might stand me in good stead at some future time. OK, so my social life will suffer to some extent, but that isn't a disaster, just a temporary inconvenience. I won't have to spend *all* my evenings working. So, I'll get on with it and not foolishly cut off my nose to spite my face.'

Once you get started on a disagreeable task, you will often find that it isn't quite as bad as you thought it would be. You tend to magnify the 'horrors' of the task before you start on it, and that, of course, easily gives you the excuse you are looking for not to do it at all!

Conclusion

The theme of this chapter has been that it makes little sense to run away from life's difficulties and responsibilities, either through procrastination or through the abuse of drugs, or both. Short-range hedonism, or the insistence on immediate gratification, is a senseless philosophy in today's world. A more sensible and ultimately more personally satisfying alternative is to adopt a harder-headed, longer-range approach to pleasure and enjoyment. You have the brains to determine the best thing to do to make life more interesting and more satisfying for you. Not that you *must*! But once you determine what is to be done, then, no matter how unpleasant it may be, do it promptly. Acquiring self-discipline may seem unduly difficult, but in the long run you will find the 'easy' or undisciplined way harder, much less rewarding and, more often than not, self-defeating. If you do not feel too emotionally

126

blocked or upset to benefit from applying the advice contained in this chapter, then try to see what you can accomplish by working hard at it. We're not saying it's easy – it isn't. But if you diligently and consistently work at applying our philosophy, you may well look back on it some day as one of the best investments you ever made. Good luck!

SUMMARY POINTS FOR CHAPTER 8

(1) Make the acquisition of self-discipline one of your top priorities in life. We're not born with it, it is a habit we have to acquire if we want to feel we are in control of our life and achieve our aims with the minimum expenditure of time and energy.

(2) If you lack self-discipline, you will find it all too easy to procrastinate and shirk responsibility for your behaviour when the inevitable hassles of life confront you with problems which can be solved only by intelligent planning and co-ordinated, goal-directed action. Poor self-discipline creates more hassles, not less.

(3) Seeking to avoid pain or discomfort by taking the route which promises instant relief is a human tendency which is probably biologically based since it has obvious survival value. But instant gratification, in today's world, of our desires frequently means a much greater amount of pain or discomfort later.

(4) Long-range hedonism – putting up with present pain for future gain – is a sensible philosophy which will give you a better chance of leading a maximally satisfying existence.

(5) The basic cause of poor self-discipline is Low Frustration Tolerance (LFT). LFT not only sustains and makes worse other kinds of emotional disturbance, but also leads to chronic procrastination and the avoidance of hard work, and encourages various kinds of 'escapism' such as over-indulgence in alcohol and other drugs.

(6) Using our familiar RET method of scientifically questioning and logically examining the beliefs underlying LFT, we identified the core belief of LFT as this: 'Life conditions must not be difficult and it is easier to avoid facing many of life's difficulties and responsibilities than to undertake more rewarding forms of self-discipline.' This idea is irrational and cannot be upheld; the consequences of believing it can be serious.

(7) The other main contributors to undisciplined behaviour and principal saboteurs of intelligent, goal-directed behaviour are self-denigration, hostility and addiction. With the A-B-C model in front of you, the irrational beliefs behind self-denigration can be

quickly identified and uprooted. Replacing them by more rational ideas will help you overcome any procrastination which may be blocking you from buckling down to accomplishing whatever task confronts you.

(8) Addictions can take several forms but the psychological aspects of addiction are anchored upon the same basic irrational beliefs as are responsible for poor self-discipline:

(a) 'I must be spared the hassles of life and it is easier to avoid than to face life's difficulties and responsibilities.'

(b) 'When life is difficult others must help me by making life easier for me. I need them to rely on.'

(c) 'Because it is preferable that I experience pleasure rather than pain, the world absolutely must arrange this and life is horrible, and I can't bear it, when the world does not.'

9

Staying Emotionally Healthy

Let us suppose that you have read and understood the principles of rational living that we have set out in this book and have begun to put them into practice. You have succeeded in changing some of your self-defeating thoughts, feelings and behaviours, and you feel good about this. You feel more in control of your life. You are less afraid to take sensible risks in going after what you want. You have had some successes; perhaps you have gone for job interviews and landed a good job; or you have done well in a love affair. You have proved to yourself that you have some executive ability, or that you have lovable ways and characteristics. Good!

Alas! Life is not an ever-onward progression towards better things, better times. There will be times, hopefully not many, when you will fall back, even far back, into some of your old irrational ways. Perhaps you thought you had your old irrational ideas and self-defeating behaviours licked once and for all. Well, it isn't as easy as that! None of us is perfect, and practically all of us take one step backwards for every two or three steps forward. It is human nature to improve a little, then to stop or even fall back a step or two before moving forward once more. When you backslide, accept it as normal, as part of your human fallibility. Don't feel ashamed or think you are weak when some of your old emotional problems return in spite of your brave efforts to overcome them. We will show you presently a number of useful ways to tackle a situation in which you find yourself beset by emotional problems similar to those you thought you had already conquered. It is important for you to realize that you have strong innate or biological tendencies to subscribe to irrational ideas, that is, to think in absolutistic, '*must*urbatory' ways. Our parents, teachers and significant others teach us cultural standards many of which are, in fact, quite sensible prescriptions about what to do and what not to do. But because, like our parents before us, we are naturally crooked thinkers, we find it easy to inflate these fairly sensible prescriptions for desirable or preferential behaviour into absolute *musts* and *necessities*. When we substitute *shoulds*, *oughts*, and *musts* for desires and preferences, then we are in trouble. The superstitions and unrealistic expectations of our culture, as portrayed in dramas and films and modelled by the mass media generally, may strongly contribute to the prevalence of irrational ideas and behaviours, but it is our own innate tendencies to think crookedly and irrationally which make these ideas stick. Fortunately, we humans also have the ability to think logically and scientifically. Although we don't regard the scientific method as infallible or sacred, it is the most efficient method we know of helping you to discover which of your beliefs are irrational and self-defeating, and how to use factual evidence and logical thinking to rid yourself of them. Let's go on now to demonstrate the effectiveness of RET techniques for dealing with emotional problems when these arise once more to trouble you.

Backsliding – and how to get back on track

How do you feel when, after a period of progress in solving your emotional problems, you once more become emotionally derailed? If your reaction is similar to that of many other people who have benefited from applying RET principles to their lives but have subsequently slipped back, you will tend to put yourself down for having allowed an old problem to arise and smite you again. It's as if you are ashamed of yourself for having displayed weakness in allowing some previously solved problem to recur and get the better of you again. Typically, you have a confrontation with someone, and instead of dealing firmly but calmly with the other person, you 'lose your rag' and end up in an angry shouting match. Or you lose the love or approval of someone who had become important to you, and you make yourself depressed. In either case, you not only experience the feelings of anger or depression, but also feel guilty or ashamed for having become enraged or depressed. You now have two problems for the price of one! You tell yourself: 'What an idiot I am for having lost my cool with so-and-so last week. After all I've learned, I *ought* to have known better!' Or, if you make yourself depressed when you lose the love or approval of some significant person, you typically berate yourself with: 'Oh *No*, I've done it again! What a fool I am for making myself depressed about something I *should* now be able to handle!'

Whenever you find yourself in a similar situation, we advise you to tackle your secondary problem first. Go after your self-denigration. Giving yourself a trouncing for permitting a previous problem to reassert itself is hardly the best way to help you get down quickly to tackling your real problem. First of all, you can assume that whatever your previous problem might have been, it became established through your habitually thinking the irrational thoughts which created it in the first place. To make something into a habit requires practice. To break a habit also requires practice. Even if you have practised a self-defeating habit (such as enraging yourself when your wishes get blocked), and practised it for many years, you can still disrupt it and substitute a more appropriate pattern of behaviour, provided you work and practise the new behaviour until it, in time, becomes your habitual behaviour. To help you achieve this, we advise you to turn your attention to three very important insights. We have discussed them in previous chapters, but we would like you to study them again until you clearly understand and remember them.

The three RET insights

Insight No. 1

You mainly *feel* the way you *think*. When unpleasant or frustrating things, or activating events, happen to you at point A, you hold two sets of beliefs about them: you hold a rational set of beliefs that lead you to feel sad, regretful or annoyed, and you also hold a set of irrational beliefs that lead you to feel anxious, depressed or self-denigrating and enraged. If you have habitually reacted to unpleasant events in your life by focusing, consciously or unconsciously, on your irrational beliefs, you will tend to act on these irrational beliefs whenever similar obnoxious things happen to you in future. The more you practise thinking irrational thoughts, the more strongly established they become. Although unpleasant events in your life, aided and abetted by social learning, encourage you to feel upset, you still largely choose to disturb yourself about these unpleasant events. We're not saying you are *totally* responsible for your emotional upsets and self-defeating behaviours; as we noted above, you are influenced to some extent by your biology, the kind of social learning you have been exposed to, and the culture you have been brought up in. Nonetheless you do, to quite a large degree, control your own emotional destiny. By and large you choose how often and how intensely you upset yourself. And to a large extent you can even choose how long to *remain* upset once you become upset. If you mainly create your emotional states, it is quite likely that you can change them.

Insight No. 2

Regardless of how or when you first acquired your irrational beliefs and your self-sabotaging habits, you still choose to believe and hold on to them today. That is why you are *now* disturbed. Your early childhood, your past history and conditioning affect you. They affected you then, and they affect you now. But they don't disturb you. You do. As a child you went along with what your parents and other early influences taught you. Lacking the critical capacity to distinguish the sensible things you were taught from the nonsense, you readily acquired a number of irrational notions about yourself and your world, the *shoulds*, *oughts* and *musts*. If you are upset today, it is because you still actively hold on to those early acquired views and still refuse to rethink and act against the irrational beliefs which you originally upset yourself with. Stop griping about your past and admit that you at least partly created your upset feelings then by the views you held then. Then the more you explore what you are *now* doing to cause your upset feelings, the more insight you will have into what's going on. We all carry around a lot of baggage acquired from the past. If you find that some of it is holding you back from living a more emotionally satisfying life – dump it! We will show you how!

Insight No. 3

In some ways, this insight no 3 is even more important than the previous two. It says that merely changing your thinking is not in itself likely to be enough to enable you to bring about a basic personality change. Rethinking your philosophy is a necessary part of the process of basic personality change, but to enable it to work effectively, you will discover that you will rarely free yourself from your 'emotional' hang-ups unless you specifically, vigorously and persistently *act* and propel yourself in directions that counteract your irrational ideas. *Acting* against your ingrained irrational notions will help you to give them up and the inappropriate feelings and self-destructive behaviours which accompany them. Suppose, for example, that you are afraid of going up to strangers at a dance and asking them to dance with you; or you are afraid of going up to perfect strangers at a cocktail party or other social events and striking up a conversation with them because you are not very good at conversation and you are afraid of being ignored, or cold-shouldered, or rejected and made to feel inadequate. Of course, you 'know' that nobody can *make* you feel anything, but if you really do know it, how come you are avoiding doing what you are afraid to do? Telling yourself, 'I know I can go up to somebody interesting – or attractive-looking and strike up a conversation, and if they turn their back on me, it won't kill me' is fine but on its own it won't help you change. Only when you actually *do* it – and not just once, but many times – will you really convince yourself that you can do these things. As long as you merely say 'I know I can' you only have evidence that you *think* you can. But once you actually *do* these things you were afraid to do, you have proof that you really *can* do them. Acting goes with thinking; they influence and interact with each other. Insight alone usually doesn't lead to behavioural change; and changing your behaviour by itself tends to lead to only limited understanding and modification of your irrational beliefs. It is the combination of changed thinking and persistent and forceful acting against your irrational fears and habits which makes effective personality change possible. Remember, your old self-defeating habits have become highly rehearsed. It follows that to disrupt them radically, and to eliminate them, you need constantly to practise their opposites.

Armed with these three RET insights, we can now proceed to show you how to tackle the re-emergence of an old problem and continue to maintain your RET gains.

Go back to basics

When an old feeling of anxiety, depression or self-deprecation returns to bother you, try to remind yourself exactly what thoughts, feelings and behaviours you once identified and changed to bring about your improvement. Think back to how you previously used the RET techniques described in this book to get over your earlier emotional disturbances. For example, you may recall that when you denigrated yourself for some failing or other, you challenged the irrational idea that you were a worthless person. Go back and rehearse the arguments you went through to convince yourself that a mistaken act or a wrong deed does not make you a bad person. Remember and apply the important RET principle of refraining from rating your *self*, your *being*, but of measuring your acts, deeds, traits and performances. Remember that you are always a *person* who behaves well or badly, but never a *good person* or a *bad person*. No matter how badly you may have fallen back and brought on your old disturbance again, you can still fully accept yourself with your weak or foolish behaviour. Then, once you have truly accepted yourself as a person who, on this occasion, has once more acted weakly, but is not a weak or inadequate person, you can then try hard to change your behaviour.

Use the three RET insights as a framework to guide you and remind you of how you identified and tackled your irrational beliefs and self-defeating behaviours in the past, and how you can continue to use these insights now and in the future. When an old, or even a new, emotional problem arises to trouble you, the framework will provide you with your bearings and help you to plot a course leading to a rational interpretation and successful resolution of your problem.

As an individual, you may be unique – but your problems and their causes, are not! Literally millions of people throughout the world have problems similar to yours, and act in similar ways to bring them on. Virtually all emotional and behavioural difficulties are created by absolutistic irrational beliefs. You, your neighbour next door, the TV presenter on your screen, the business tycoon, politicians, preachers and generals the world over, all experience emotional hang-ups and behavioural or personality problems at some time in their lives. Indeed, some of them appear to have them throughout their *entire* lives! Whatever your (and their) irrational beliefs are, they can be overcome only by strongly and persistently disputing and acting against them. You tend to have three major kinds of irrational belief which create and sustain your emotional and behavioural problems. We have already gone into them in previous chapters but, in view of their importance, we make no apology for returning to them here.

Irrational Belief No. 1

'I *must* do well and win the approval of people who are important to me.' If you believe this, you will feel anxious and depressed and hate yourself. You will feel anxious when you think 'What if I don't do well, as I *must*!', and if you actually fail to do well and win the approval of someone important to you, you conclude, 'Because I am not doing as well as I *must*, I am an inadequate and worthless nobody!' And you also conclude, 'Since I have failed to win the approval of someone I deemed important to me, as I simply *had* to, it's *awful* and *terrible*!' Your 'awfulizing' here will lead you towards depression. And you then follow up your 'awfulizing' with 'Because I *absolutely should not* have failed and been rejected, I'll *always* fail and be rejected! I'll *never* be accepted, as I *must*, so my life is just wasted and I'll *never* be happy again!' This over-generalizing and self-pity, together with your 'awfulizing', is all you need to push you into a depressed state.

Can you see how self-defeating this belief is? So long as you convince yourself that you *must* succeed at important tasks, and *have to* be approved or loved by significant people in your life, then when you fail – as you probably will, at times – to win someone's love or approval, you will almost inevitably make yourself anxious and depressed instead of sorry and frustrated.

Irrational Belief No. 2

'Other people, especially those I love, *must* treat me fairly and considerately!' It would be lovely if everybody treated us fairly and considerately at all times. But how long do you think it will be before they don't? Not very long! If you subscribe to this irrational idea, it won't be long before you make yourself angry. For you will conclude: 'Because others are not treating me as fairly and considerately as they *absolutely should*, they are rotten people and deserve to be condemned and punished!' This irrational idea, like the first, simply bears no relation to the facts of human fallibility. People are people, and there is no law of the universe which says that they must treat us nicely or behave any differently than they actually do. No matter how desirable consideration of others may be, it doesn't *have to* exist. There are no 'have to's in the universe.

Irrational Belief No. 3

'The conditions under which I live *must* be comfortable and free from major hassles!' There are innumerable variations on this theme. One is: 'I *must* get what I want quickly and easily, without having to work too hard to get it.' Another is: 'I *must* avoid, rather than face and deal with, many of life's difficulties and responsibilities because I *need* immediate comfort and it's too hard to discipline myself to put up with present pain to achieve future gain.' A third is: 'I *must* continue to suffer endlessly if I have handicaps. If I have a serious handicap, I can do practically nothing to overcome it, and life is so unfair and *horrible* when I am so handicapped that it is hardly worth living!' With any of these beliefs you will tend to create feelings of resentment, apathy, depression, alienation, self-pity, and possibly feelings of anger and hostility as well.

You will have realized that this irrational idea and its variants not only create these emotional disturbances we've just mentioned, but also lead to several self-defeating behaviours which you have already come across: low frustration tolerance (LFT, or, to give it its technical name, discomfort anxiety); procrastination; avoidance of responsibility; and withdrawal. Of course it is unfair and unfortunate if you are born with a handicap. And, of course, it is too bad when the conditions under which you live are hard, uncomfortable and full of hassles. But where is it written that life *must* be easy, that fairness *must* reign upon this earth and that justice and equality *must* be made available to all? If life *had* to be like that, it would be! OK, maybe human ingenuity, plus a goodly amount of blood, sweat and tears, will create a better world for us some day. But we don't run the universe; and while the conditions under which we live may improve somewhat, it is highly unlikely they will ever become ideal. Life is spelt H-A-S-S-L-E!

You will sometimes hear folk declare, 'I can't stand it!' when some misfortune assails them, or when their goals are frustrated. Obviously, they *can* stand 'it', or they would cease to exist. You can stand anything until you die. You may not like your particular lot, but whining about it won't help make it better and most likely will encourage you to feel even more miserable. Instead, sensibly figure out what you can do to minimize your pain and discomfort and increase your pleasure. At the same time, vigorously counterattack the absolutistic *shoulds, oughts* and *musts* which you bring to your frustrating or obnoxious conditions and upset yourself with. Actively work against your LFT; regard it as a challenge to enjoy life while working hard with your RET insights to upset yourself only minimally even though you have to accept a certain amount of hassle and deprivation in your life.

Replace your demands with your desires

Armed with the three main irrational beliefs, you may now appreciate that irrational ideas are part and parcel of your everyday repertoire of thoughts and feelings and that you employ them, consciously or unconsciously, in a considerable variety of situations. Whenever you feel seriously upset, or find yourself behaving in a distinctly self-defeating manner, realize that you are holding and acting upon one or more of these irrational beliefs. If you have been successful at identifying and disputing the irrational beliefs creating your emotional upset in one situation, you can extend the same principle to any other situation where you have an emotional problem. Realize that it is almost impossible to disturb yourself and to remain disturbed in *any* way if you really give up your absolutistic demands – your dogmatic *shoulds*, *oughts* and *musts* – and replace them with flexible desires and preferences. Strong desires and preferences are healthy. They won't get you into trouble as long as you refuse to escalate them into dire necessities.

Incidentally, watch your language! What this means is that if instead of saying 'I *must* do well and be approved' you merely change your language to 'I *prefer* to do well and be approved', you will only be fooling yourself if what you still really believe is, 'But I really *have to* do well and *have got to* be approved'. Changing your language does not necessarily mean that you have changed your thinking! Changing your thinking is not quite so easy as that. In fact, it isn't easy at all; it requires persistent work and practice at disputing your irrational beliefs until you clearly see that they are untrue or unprovable and cannot be rationally supported. How will you know when you have truly given them up? Only when your feelings of disturbance truly disappear will you have succeeded in really convincing yourself of the truth of your rational answers. Even then, don't stop disputing! Continue to dispute your irrational beliefs over and over again until your rational answers become hardened and habitual. Just as you build up your body muscles by constant exercise, so, too, can you develop intellectual and emotional muscle by continually finding and actively and vigorously disputing your irrational beliefs. If you only superficially convince yourself of your new rational philosophy, it won't help you very much or persist very long. That is why some people fall back after improving emotionally. If you fall back after achieving some initial improvement, don't castigate or denigrate yourself for your lapse. Instead, get back to the drawing board! Go after those irrational beliefs you only half laid to rest and dispute them strongly and vigorously over and over again until you convince yourself and really feel you can say, 'I do not *need* what I *want*. I never *have* to succeed, no matter how strongly I *wish* to! I *can* stand being rejected by someone I care for. It won't *kill* me – I can *still* lead a happy life! *No* human is damnable and worthless, and that especially includes *me*!'

Act against your irrational beliefs

Remember the importance of *acting* against your irrational ideas. If you feel uncomfortable in forcing yourself to do things that you are afraid to try, don't give yourself relief by opting out. If you allow yourself to avoid doing something you consider risky in order to avoid the discomfort of doing it, you'll preserve your discomfort forever! It is often a good idea to make yourself as uncomfortable as you can in order to eradicate your irrational fears about doing this 'risky' thing and so lose your anxiety and discomfort later.

Similarly with procrastination: do what needs to be done fast! Don't sit and think about it until it is too late to do anything effective. If you experience difficulty in getting going, reward yourself with certain things you enjoy *after* you have completed the task you were inclined to avoid. If rewarding yourself doesn't work, give yourself a severe penalty – such as giving a large sum of money to some cause you detest, or spending two hours of your time talking to some person you find exceptionally boring – every time you procrastinate. You will find that tackling the avoided task is not so bad by comparison!

Monitor your progress

You can monitor your progress from time to time. Did you know that change for the better can be measured? Well, it can. Suppose, for illustration, that you have previously had a problem controlling your tendency to outbursts of anger directed against your spouse. You've acquired some insight into how you create your own anger through reading this book and putting into practice our advice. So far so good. But occasionally you still fly into a rage when your spouse behaves towards you in a manner you consider to be uncaring and neglectful. You can measure your progress in overcoming your angry outbursts along three dimensions: *frequency*, *intensity* and *duration*. In other words, you can ask yourself, for example, *how often* you now enrage yourself when your mate acts inconsiderately towards you compared to, say, three months ago, before you began to understand the real cause of your angry episodes. Similarly, you can ask yourself *how intensely* you anger yourself nowadays compared to the past when you thought it was the way your spouse carried on that upset you. Finally, whenever you do get angry over your mate's behaviour, you can ask yourself how long you remain in an angry mood. If you can answer honestly 'Less often! Less intensely! Less long!' you can assume you have made some real progress. Your aim, of course, would be to reach the stage when you can answer 'Very rarely!' or 'Not at all!' So keep trying! You've nothing to lose except your high blood pressure or ulcers!

Change your inappropriate feelings but not your appropriate feelings

We attach great importance in RET to teaching people to distinguish between their *appropriate* feelings and their *inappropriate* feelings. This is no mere semantic quibble. Let us once more try to make clear to you this very important point. RET is alone in clearly distinguishing appropriate from inappropriate feelings. Usually, we deal with people's inappropriate *negative* feelings since negative feelings are more commonly encountered among people with emotional disturbance than inappropriate positive feelings. Nevertheless, positive feelings of an exaggerated or inappropriate kind also carry distinct disadvantages. We will consider both negative and positive feelings here for completeness. Our aim is to try to make clear the difference for the purpose of helping you stay emotionally healthy.

When you go after something important you want, such as a good job or an attractive love partner, and you fail to get what you want, you may create both appropriate and inappropriate negative feelings. We consider your strong feelings of sadness, irritation and concern to be healthy and appropriate for two reasons. First, having strong desires and striving to reach your goals is likely to promote your survival. If you had no desires whatever, you would tend to neglect your health, fail to eat nourishing food and probably die of some ailment. Second, appropriate feelings help you to *express* your displeasure when undesirable things happen to you and motivate you to work at changing them.

However, we define as inappropriate and harmful any feelings of depression, anxiety, anger, or self-hatred which you may experience, and again there are two reasons why. First, they stem from your unrealistic commands that unpleasant or unfortunate events absolutely *must* not exist. Second, they will usually interfere with and block your ability to change these events when they do happen to exist.

Thus, if you feel sad and concerned when you are passed over after applying for that job you very much wanted, you will try to determine what factors were against you and how you could change them and strengthen your chances of being accepted another time. But if you become depressed or over-concerned about ever getting another chance of a good job, you will spend so much of your time obsessed with this possibility that your confidence will suffer and your standard of performance in your present job may fall to such an extent as to seriously jeopardize your chance of getting any other job.

Similarly, if you are appropriately saddened and disappointed about being rejected by a love partner, especially after the relationship had been going well from the beginning and you had experienced reciprocation for a time, you may be quite strongly motivated to discover why you were abandoned, and to win back that person's love. Or if you think that is no longer an option, you may try to find another more suitable partner. On the other hand, if you inappropriately become angry with your rejector, giving vent to your anger will most likely drive him or her away and ruin your chances of ever getting back together again. Or if you become depressed and full of self-hatred over your being rejected you will tend to withdraw completely from meeting or encountering other possible partners and almost guarantee that you will never win the kind of relationship you want. In other words, inappropriate negative feelings such as panic, depression or rage will interfere with your ability to cope effectively with your problems and to improve the quality of your life.

Once you realize that you cause your own psychologically unhealthy feelings by believing strongly in some dogmatic *should*, *ought* or *must*, and that you are capable of changing your inappropriate (*musturbatory*) feelings back into preferences and desires, through challenging and uprooting these shoulds, oughts and musts, you are well on the way to regaining emotional control of your life.

Now let's look at the difference between your appropriate and inappropriate *positive* feelings. Joy is normally a fine and healthy feeling. Suppose you have done exceptionally well in some area of your life. Let's say you have won an exceptionally good job against really stiff competition, coming out top against several hundred competing candidates. You feel very happy. But are you happy and delighted about your performance? Of course. But is that all? It certainly is appropriate to feel quite elated about having done so well; but aren't you also extending that great feeling about your outstanding performance to *you*, *yourself*? If so, you are not the first! Just as you sometimes rate yourself as a bad or stupid person when you act immorally or stupidly, so, too, you sometimes rate yourself as a great and noble person when you act outstandingly well, as, for example, when you pull off a triumph of some sort. In other words, you jump from 'My behaviour is outstanding' to 'I am therefore an outstanding person!' We call this an inappropriate positive feeling because you grandiosely rate yourself above other people. Can you see that it is just as illegitimate to label yourself as a good or noble person when you behave well, as it is to rate yourself as a wicked or stupid person when you behave badly? Evaluating your *self* or *being* on the basis of your acts and performances will almost certainly get you into an emotional tangle, because when you don't perform outstandingly well the next time you set out to equal your previous performance, you drop back to denigrating yourself for having done badly. Be happy about your fine performances but don't deify yourself for your achievements. A string of successes does not make you a fine and worthy individual any more than a succession of failures makes you an unworthy or useless person. Once again, look for your *shoulds* and *musts*. You don't *have to* do well, and you don't *need* people to view you as a marvellous person in order to accept yourself and be happy with your life. If you think you absolutely *have to* do well to win the approval of others, you will make yourself anxious about later falling on your face and disappointing those others who previously admired you.

If you bring on any of these inappropriate feelings, look for the demands with which you create them and work at disputing them until you actually do change your disturbed feelings to more appropriate ones. Read and reread this book until you know it thoroughly! If you occasionally lapse back into your old emotional upsets, refuse to make yourself even more upset by denigrating yourself for it. Go back to the drawing board and calmly but determinedly seek out the irrational ideas with which you have upset yourself. Be assured, they are there! And when you find them, uproot them using the various thinking, feeling and action techniques we have tried to teach you. And don't give up until you really feel better. Then continue to use them on a daily basis until they become truly established as a part of your psychological make-up.

Become creatively absorbed

Most intelligent and perceptive people rarely feel particularly happy remaining inert for long periods of time. A life of passive enjoyment tends to become boring for people who are accustomed to using their grey matter and who find striving actively for what they want out of life to be much more satisfying. As active goal-orientated people ourselves, we strongly espouse becoming vitally absorbed in some long-range goals and purposes in life. Keeping oneself goal-orientated for the rest of one's days is, we are convinced on the basis of our experience, one of the very best ways of enjoying life and staying emotionally healthy.

One of the most vital forms of absorption is loving. Giving love can be a creative, self-expressing kind of involvement in some person or some thing outside yourself. You can be creatively absorbed in loving other people, you can love animals, you can love things such as works of art, or antiques, and you can be lovingly absorbed in ideas or philosophizing. Giving love can be more satisfying in the long term than being loved. It's nice to be loved, of course, but being loved can sometimes become a little restricting if your lover is too demanding of your time and company. On the other hand, giving love offers you almost unlimited scope to express to the full your imagination and creativity towards the loved person or thing without the restricting ties you may experience from a monopolizing or over-demanding lover. Living essentially means doing, creating, thinking, loving. You cancel it out when you allow yourself to become inert, passive, or inhibited and hence tend to lose out in getting truly absorbed in living your life to the full.

It is certainly not part of our brief to tell you *what* to do with your life. You are a unique individual, biologically and socially, and only you can decide what you would most like to do, and what would bring you the most pleasure and satisfaction. We, the authors of this book, know what we are aiming to do, and what turns us on and what doesn't. If you don't really know yet what you might undertake in the way of a truly absorbing activity, try to find out by experiment. We can't tell you what to try out, but we can offer you a little advice on *how* to find out.

You know already some of the things you find interesting and enjoyable. But what else might you find enjoyable? What about trying new and different foods? You might think, 'Oh, I know I wouldn't like that!' but how do you know until you try it? Or, have you tried introducing yourself to interesting strangers and finding out what they truly enjoy and actively involve themselves in? Some of their enthusiasms may be the very thing for you. Try to find things to do that you will still enjoy many years hence. You might have loved hockey in your youth, but sports that involve lots of physical exertion may be impractical in your later life.

Remember that you do have a limited life span and can cram only so many things into your twenty-four-hour day. As we have already pointed out, life is full of hassles and it is important to accept this reality. But if you push yourself without complaint to do the various onerous tasks you find necessary to do in order to enjoy the more satisfying things you have chosen in life, you will not mind the inconveniences so much. As long as you are alive, the only thing you can ever lose in life is pleasure. You have a right to happiness, so make that your goal. You live because you live, and there appears to be no special reason or purpose for your existence. You may invent one if you wish, but you can't prove it. You have the right to define your own basic goals and purposes.

What are some of the major life goals or purposes you might pursue? You could resolve to develop your artistic abilities – become a painter, musician, or sculptor. Or, if you are socially minded you might undertake some kind of community service. For example, you could join a team set up to help people in the developing countries to harness their countries' resources to their best advantage. Or, if you are deeply religious, you could become a missionary or evangelist and try to secure a more general acceptance of your ideals. Or, if you love animals, you could devote your life to caring for them, especially abandoned or sick pets, by establishing an animal sanctuary. Or, you could become a business tycoon and aim to head a multinational corporation.

Whatever your aims – be they some form of community service, developing your creative potential, animal welfare, or the pursuit of money, power and romantic love – you will find the RET principles set forth in this book of considerable help in cutting through your emotional problems and achieving your personal and vocational goals with minimum stress and maximum satisfaction.

As with most other aspects of living, you can only discover what truly interests or excites you by open-mindedly experimenting with as many possibilities as you have time for and can reasonably afford. Some of the things you enjoy may be self-defeating or harmful to others; in which case you'd better give them up. Be idiosyncratic if that is your bent, but acting anti-socially or inconsiderately towards others will, in all probability, defeat your own ends sooner or later. Be sensibly self-interested rather than *selfish* or self-centred.

Enlightened self-interest

It is important to appreciate that in RET, selfishness means the exclusive pursuit of one's own interests while cynically disregarding the interests and aims of others. When you self-centredly push your own interests to the fore while making clear that you don't really care for anyone else's rights, your obnoxious behaviour will tend to rebound upon you, since those others whose rights you trample on will often retaliate in kind.

Enlightened self-interest, by contrast, includes an acknowledgement that we live in a social world in which others, too, have the right to pursue their own interests even if these interests are sometimes antithetical to our own. From a long-term perspective, we give priority to pursuing our own most important goals since it is likely that other people will do the same. That is to say, they will put their own interest first, just as we do ours.

You can rationally put others' interests before your own *some* of the time and lovingly sacrifice yourself for selected others whether or not you believe they will treat you equally well in return. But don't let it become a continuing habit! Some of those for whom you sacrifice yourself will respond lovingly and considerately but others will not. Some will exploit your kindness, while many more, those who are ignorant or emotionally disturbed, will be unable to treat you, or indeed anyone else, morally or fairly.

By all means, then, sacrifice yourself to some degree for those loved ones and those for whom you care, but not overwhelmingly or totally. Accept responsibility for running your own life. Unless you are severely handicapped in some way, you do not need massive support from others, nor is it rational to demand it. You act morally towards others when you protect the rights of others, because in that way you abet social survival and help to create the kind of world in which you yourself can live comfortably and happily.

Conclusion

This final chapter has been something of a 'booster', designed to remind you of some of the more important points you need to learn in order to live a happier, more fulfilling life. Making yourself miserable about anything is unreasonable; you not only prevent yourself from achieving your potential for a sane and happy life by becoming over-concerned or extremely agitated when confronted with life's many hassles, but you also become a bit of a pain in the neck to those you associate with. Thus you needlessly defeat yourself and obtain much less of what you want than is actually available.

Most people today seem to be beset by sex, love and other problems and have a difficult time in trying to behave with at least a modicum of rationality in this none too rational world. While it is gratifying that more and more people are taking their problems to trained professionals, many more seem to be content to consult soothsayers, astrologers, preachers and other sources whose competence and qualifications in the counselling field are questionable. Still other people prefer to talk things over with their physician. These days, however, most GPs have little time to sit and listen to problems of a non-medical nature. For some of these people, ventilating their emotional problems may help them acquire a new perspective and start them on the road to some improvement. But more often it won't. Talking by itself is usually *not enough*, as you will have appreciated by now. The Samaritans are well known for providing a 'listening ear' and have probably helped many troubled people along the route to greater self-acceptance. The trouble is that people who accept themselves only after they see that someone else, such as the Samaritan, accepts them, tend to become dependent on a regular 'sympathy fix', and, as our Samaritan contacts will confirm, become habitual callers over long periods of time. So long as they have a sympathetic ear to listen to their troubles, they are seemingly content, but the problems themselves remain and are unlikely to go away. If you have a problem with yourself or your relationships which you feel unable to resolve through your own efforts, by all means seek professional help, preferably from a counsellor trained in RET or someone experienced in the cognitive behaviour therapy field. You can still use this book to supplement and reinforce the gains you obtain from personal counselling.

Some of your friends and associates can probably use the main teachings of RET just as you can. Don't hesitate to encourage them to read this book and discuss with you some of the main points we have presented in these pages. The more effectively your lovers, friends and relatives can cope with their lives and their emotional problems, the more mutually enjoyable will your contact be with them. Not that we are guaranteeing you, or anyone else, abiding happiness! As we have been at pains to point out, there are no guarantees in the universe. Moreover, you would do well to look after your physical health as well as your emotional health. Find a sensible diet that suits you and stick to it. Take regular exercise and get adequate rest and relaxation.

Finally, actively work at and *practise* the new philosophy we have tried to teach you in these pages until it becomes easy and 'natural' for you to follow. It's not easy. In fact, it's very hard to do what we are encouraging you to do, at least for the first few weeks or months you first work at it. Don't give up! In the long run it's much harder *not* to change your old irrational ideas and self-destructive or inhibiting habits; *and* it will be much harder that way *forever*. It's your choice. If your basic philosophy is that of taking charge of your own life and running it as sensibly as you can and being happy in spite of the innumerable pitfalls and troubles that are likely to beset you, you have an excellent chance of living a spirited, even a joyful life, in this up-and-down world of ours. What's more, you'll have a better chance of contributing some improvement to the world and eventually leaving it a better place than you found it. Why not try it and see? Good luck!

SUMMARY POINTS FOR CHAPTER 9

(1) Staying emotionally healthy doesn't come about automatically. It requires continuous work and practice to make the new philosophy

you are trying to acquire into an integral part of your life. Old habits of thinking and behaviour don't just melt effortlessly away. They will occasionally reassert themselves, temporarily wresting control from the newer and more desirable ways of thinking and feeling you have begun to achieve.

(2) Whenever you find yourself slipping back into the old habits you thought you had abandoned for good, or when some old emotional problem returns to plague you, don't feel ashamed or dejected. Accept it as normal, as part of your human fallibility. We all have innate tendencies to think in absolutistic, *musturbatory* ways; we are naturally crooked thinkers, it comes easy to us! So what do we do? Go back to basics.

(3) Any previous problem you may have had became established through your habitually thinking the irrational thoughts which created it to start with. Right? OK, go after those irrational beliefs and reconvince yourself of their falseness. If you are denigrating yourself for having slipped back, tackle your self-denigration first. Then, after you really see how needless that is, you can go on to tackle head on your earlier problem, using the various techniques we have been teaching in this book.

(4) To help you do an even better job of tackling that old emotional problem which has raised its ugly head again, carefully go over again the three RET insights and keep going over them until you really understand them. These insights provide you with an excellent framework to regain your bearings and help you to plot a course leading to a successful resolution of your problem. Any new emotional problem you may experience can be dealt with in the same efficient way.

(5) Repeat and study carefully the three main irrational beliefs. Understand why they are irrational and why they cannot be accepted as true. See how many variations of these three irrational beliefs you can come up with and remember them. Keep looking for your absolutistic demands on yourself and others, the *shoulds*, *oughts* and *musts*, and replace them with flexible, non-dogmatic desires and preferences.

(6) *Act* against your irrational ideas until you become comfortable doing things you previously were afraid to try. Use self-management techniques (Chapter 2), Rational-Emotive Imagery (Chapter 5) and shame-attacking exercises (Chapter 7) to put muscle into your newly acquired RET philosophies.

(7) Monitor your progress and convince yourself that you really can make headway against even your most stubborn self-defeating habits.

(8) Practise distinguishing between your appropriate and inappropriate feelings and understand why the difference is important. Realise that your inappropriate feelings stem from your strong dogmatic shoulds, oughts and musts and that, through challenging and uprooting these shoulds, oughts and musts, you will be well on your way to regaining emotional control of your life.

(9) Become creatively absorbed in some long-range goal or project. Vital absorption in some activity is healthy and helps promote your survival and personal happiness. The various RET thinking, feeling and action techniques we have taught you will be of considerable help to you in achieving whatever goals you set yourself in life. If you wish to remain emotionally healthy and to direct your own life confidently, keep practising these RET techniques on a daily basis until they become truly established as a part of your psychological make-up. You will benefit not only yourself but also your loved ones. And you may well leave the world a saner, happier place than you found it.